Therapeutic Approaches in Common Obstetrics and Gynecological Disorders

Inositols

Guide to Practical Applications in Obstetrics and Gynecology

THERAPEUTIC APPROACHES IN COMMON OBSTETRICS AND GYNECOLOGICAL DISORDERS

VITTORIO UNFER - SERIES EDITOR

A.G.UN.CO OBSTETRICS AND GYNECOLOGY CENTER, ROME, ITALY

Inositols: Guide to Practical Applications in Obstetrics and Gynecology

Vittorio Unfer (Editor)

2019. ISBN: 978-1-53614-912-8 (Hardcover)
2019. ISBN: 978-1-53614-913-5 (e-Book)

Alpha Lipoic Acid: New Perspectives and Clinical Use in Obstetrics and Gynecology

Vittorio Unfer (Editor)

2018. ISBN: 978-1-53613-592-3 (Hardcover)
2018. ISBN: 978-1-53613-593-0 (e-Book)

THERAPEUTIC APPROACHES IN COMMON OBSTETRICS AND GYNECOLOGICAL DISORDERS

INOSITOLS

GUIDE TO PRACTICAL APPLICATIONS IN OBSTETRICS AND GYNECOLOGY

VITTORIO UNFER
EDITOR

nova
Medicine & Health
New York

NOTICE TO THE READER

Library of Congress Cataloging-in-Publication Data

ISBN: 978-1-53614-912-8
Library of Congress Control Number: 2019931117

Published by Nova Science Publishers, Inc. † New York

CONTENTS

FOREWORD

Inositols, a family of simple carbohydrates naturally found in several foods (cereals, nuts, fruits), are concentrated in the phospholipids layer of our cells. They are bioactive compounds with structural similarities to glucose and are involved in cellular signaling. Among the nine stereoisomers, two predominates in eukaryotic cells, myo-inositol (MI) and D-chiro-inositol (DCI).

Both MI and DCI are involved in physiological functions and have been used for diverse therapeutic aims, in some cases exploiting their feature to exist in different enantiomeric forms, each one with specific tasks.

Since an increasing number of researches and investigations have been realized on inositol(s) properties, pathological conditions caused by their imbalance and finally their possible clinical use, it is essential to reaffirm and examine in-depth a few points on this matter.

Therefore, in this book the effort of the authors is to address all the possible theoretical and practical applications of these molecules in obstetrics and gynecology.

Overall, chapters of this book reported that inositols properties are susceptible of pharmacological exploitment, namely regulating various metabolic pathways and hormonal signaling, allowing proposals of therapeutic application.

Specifically, there is coverage (and a confirmation) of the efficacy of nutritional inositols in correcting endocrine and metabolic alterations in women affected by Polycystic Ovary Syndrome. Accordingly, the therapeutic role of inositols is described also as far as the removal of reproductive failures in case of insulin-resistance related disorders.

Some new information is present as far as pregnancy is concerned. Indeed, the improved metabolism in the mother induced by inositol supplement, is associated with a prevention of gestational diabetes. Such ameliorated intrauterine environment is accompanied by significant changes in the cardiovascular activity of the offspring. Thus, according to experimental paradigm, it seems that inositols could be one of the way able to stop the vicious circle of the transgenerational transmission of the metabolic syndrome.

A further new potential application of inositols could arise from their activity that enables the remodeling of cytoskeleton architecture and therefore modulate the cell-microenvironment relationships.

In addition to confirm and better define the use of inositols in reproductive issues, this book offers new experimental data representing the bases for exploratory clinical research and enlarge the potential of these compounds in Obstetrics and Gynecology.

Professor Fabio Facchinetti
Mother Infant Department
University of Modena and Reggio Emilia

Modena, August 13th, 2018

PREFACE

This book offers a valuable mine of clinical information for health professionals and researchers. It gives an overview of the critical role played by Inositols in the therapeutic approach to common obstetrics and gynecological disorders. Inositols are a family of simple carbohydrates naturally found in several foods and human cells. There are potentially nine stereoisomers of Inositols, among them being myo-inositol (MI) and, to a lesser extent, D-chiro-inositol (DCI). These are the most important isoforms for the physiological processes in humans. They exert different actions in the control of glucose homeostasis: MI regulates the activation of glucose transporters and glucose utilization, while DCI modulates the glycogen synthesis. Once incorporated into phosphoglycans, they act as second messengers involved in the signaling transduction cascade of insulin. The metabolism of Inositols is dysregulated in patients with Polycystic Ovary Syndrome (PCOS), highlighting the crucial link between insulin resistance and inositol deficiency in PCOS patients. Therefore, several pre-clinical and clinical studies have been carried out to evaluate their therapeutic usefulness in pathologies where there is an imbalance in MI and DCI levels (from PCOS and gestational diabetes mellitus to infertility). The clinical evidence has demonstrated that MI can be considered widely safe and well tolerated, giving prominence to this versatile molecule. In several trials, the beneficial effect of MI in improving the metabolic and endocrine profile of women with PCOS has been highlighted extensively. Further analyses have shown that the physiological MI:DCI ratio (40:1) is the optimal approach for improving oocyte follicular development and oocyte maturation as well as ovary stimulation and pregnancy outcomes in *in vitro* fertilization (IVF) procedures. Furthermore, the reader is introduced to a broader area encompassing the Inositols scenery from the history to Inositols nutritional importance, the therapeutic use in preeclampsia, gynecologic oncology, fetal programming as well as their resistance and substance interaction. All these interesting topics will be discussed and deepened in the present book, giving the opportunity to explore in detail every aspect of this effective molecule, bringing the instructions from this guide to everyday practice.

ACKNOWLEDGMENT

Throughout this book Inositol plays a pivotal role, being the protagonist in each chapter. The book cover represents Inositol depicted as a turtle. The image was captured from an original painting realized by Mrs. Anna Finelli from Ravenna. The painting was requested by Professor Vittorio Unfer inspired by the scientific article: "*Turtles All the Way: Reflections on myo-Inositol*" by Bernard W. Agranoff (2009). The painting is currently hung in Professor Unfer office, who acknowledges the artist, Anna Finelli, for the ability in illustrating the Inositol molecule in such elegant and suggestive way.

In: Inositols
Editor: Vittorio Unfer

ISBN: 978-1-53614-912-8

Chapter 1

USE OF INOSITOLS IN GYNECOLOGY AND OBSTETRICS: A HISTORICAL OVERVIEW

Beatrice Orrù*[1]*, PhD and Vittorio Unfer*[2,*]*, MD
[1]Medical Affairs Department, Lo.Li. Pharma, Rome, Italy
[2]A.G.UN.CO Obstetrics and Gynecology Center, Rome, Italy

ABSTRACT

Inositol is a carbocyclic polyol compound ubiquitous across most life forms. Myo-inositol (MI) and D-chiro-inositol (DCI) are the two main stereisomers present in the human body. MI is synthesized endogenously from glucose 6-phosphate, and it is found at the level of cell membranes as phosphatidylinositol, bound to membrane phospholipids. It regulates the activity of several hormones such as insulin, thyroid-stimulating hormone and stimulating follicle hormone. MI is converted into DCI by an insulin dependent epimerase. They exert different activities, MI promoting glucose uptake, while DCI providing glycogen synthesis. Polycistic Ovary Syndrome is a metabolic and hormonal disorder common among women of reproductive age, linked to insulin resistance, hyperinsulinaemia and hyperandrogenism. The insulin sensitizing effects of MI and/or DCI have

* Corresponding Author's Email: vunfer@gmail.com.

been thoroughly studied, however a lot still needs to be done. The physiological ratio of these two isomers is 40:1 (MI:DCI) that has been shown to be an optimal approach for the treatment of PCOS disorders.

Keywords: inositol, myo-inositol, d-chiro-inositol, polycystic ovary syndrome, PCOS, oocytes quality

INTRODUCTION

The history of inositol is quite complex and appealing. In 1850, Johann Joseph Scherer isolated from the muscle a hexahydroxycyclohexane that he named Inositol [from Ancient Greek stem of ἰς (is, in-, "sinew, fiber"), -ose (indicating a carbohydrate), -ite ("ester"), -ol ("an alcohol")] (Irvine 2016, Majumder and Biswas 2006, Scherer 1850). Since then, this discovery has raised interest on inositol and its derivatives. In 1887, its cyclohexanol structure was established by Maquenne, who fully purified inositol from leaves (Maquenne 1887a, b, c). Nine possible stereoisomeric forms may occur subsequently to the epimerization of the six OH- groups: cis-, epi, allo-, myo-, neo-, scyllo-, L-chiro-, D-chiro- and muco- ins (Murthy 2006). Among them, myo-inositol (MI) is virtually ubiquitous in nature and is the most abundant isomer found (Wang, Safar, and Zopf 1990). Inositol can be synthesized endogenously from glucose 6-phosphate or sourced from dietary intake such as beans, citrus fruits, and whole grains (Clements and Darnell 1980). It is considered a prebiotic molecule for its great stability and its fundamental functions (Agranoff 2009).

During the following years, researchers worldwide have extended the investigation to the concentration of MI in different organs and tissues. Eisenberg and Bolden in 1964 found that testes were rich in free inositol (Eisenberg and Bolden 1964, Eisenberg, Bolden, and Loewus 1964). Further studies demonstrated high levels of inositol as well in the prostate, the epididymis and the seminal vesicles (Ghafoorunissa 1976, Lewin and Beer 1973, Voglmayr and Amann 1973). The seminal fluid is one of the richest sources of inositol with a nearly triple concentration compared to that found in plasma (Spector and Lorenzo 1975b, a). In the late eighties, Larner investigated the intracellular mediators of insulin action in order to identify a potential pharmaceutical product for treating diabetic diseases. Larner first proposed the existence of multiple mediators of insulin action suggesting that after the binding of insulin with its receptor the second step could evolve in different pathways, depending on the stimulated mediator. In 1988, he concluded that MI and D-chiro-inositol (DCI) are chemical mediators of insulin, acting through different mechanisms (Larner et al. 1988).

MI is a component of membrane-incorporated phosphatidylinositols as lipid-anchored proteins, the precursors for the second messenger's inositol-tri-phosphate and diacylglycerol. MI acts as a second messenger regulating the activity of hormones among which follicle-stimulating hormone (FSH), thyroid-stimulating hormone (TSH) and insulin (Bizzarri et al. 2016). The activation of glucose transporters and glucose utilization are controlled by MI whereas the glycogen synthesis is regulated by DCI (Heimark, McAllister, and Larner 2014, Huang et al. 1993, Larner et al. 1988, Sun et al. 2002). Both molecules are therefore able to exert an insulin-sensitizing effect reducing the circulating insulin levels. DCI is converted from MI through an insulin-dependent epimerization process (Pak et al. 1992). In diabetic mice a reduced activity of the epimerase was found, causing a deficiency of DCI and, consequently, insulin resistance suggesting that hyperinsulinemia in insulin-resistant mice could depend on the reduced epimerase activity (Sun et al. 2002). The conversion rate MI to DCI is impaired in patients with diagnosed Polycystic Ovary Syndrome (PCOS) due to insulin resistance; this aberration has been found to be exacerbated when having first-degree diabetic relatives (Genazzani et al. 2014, Larner 2002). Indeed, the familial predisposition or the pathology itself antagonizes the epimerase activity, triggering the onset of insulin resistance and compensatory hyperinsulinaemia (61). Indeed, lower levels of DCI minimize the availability of inositolphosphoglycans thus contributing to insulin resistance (Baillargeon et al. 2006). An increase of DCI urinary excretion was demonstrated in PCOS women respect to normal controls by Baillargeon and Nestler (2006). They observed a reduction of plasma DCI levels but not in MI concentration (Baillargeon and Nestler 2006).

THE LINK WITH PCOS

In the same years an association between insulin resistance and consequent hyperinsulinemia with PCOS was established (Dunaif 1997, Dunaif et al. 1989). PCOS is a health problem that affects up to 15% of the total female population in reproductive age, firstly described by Drs. Stein and Leventhal in 1935 (Stein and Leventhal 1935). It is linked to ovarian dysfunction, menstrual irregularity, metabolic and hormonal impairments. It is the most common cause of infertility (Palomba et al. 2015, Qin et al. 2013) psychological distress (Hadjiconstantinou et al. 2017), obesity (Lim et al. 2012) and it can contribute to long-term health problems like diabetes (Dunaif et al. 1989, Ehrmann et al. 1999, Legro et al. 1999) and heart disease (de Groot et al. 2011, Dunaif et al. 1989, Rizzo et al. 2009). Over the years, the presence of insulin receptors in the ovaries was shown, indicating a role for this peptide in the regulation of their function (Jarrett et al. 1985, Poretsky et al. 1985, Poretsky et al. 1984). In women with PCOS was observed that insulin directly prompts androgen production by ovarian stroma (Barbieri et al. 1986). Furthermore, in rat ovarian theca cells was shown that insulin and insulin-like growth factor I increase luteinizing hormone-stimulated androgen biosynthesis (Cara et al. 1990, Cara and Rosenfield 1988). Insulin has been shown to play an important role in the pathogenesis of PCOS, both directly and indirectly. In fact, it reduces the hepatic synthesis of the sex hormone-binding globulin, causing an increase in circulating free testosterone. DeClue et al. suggested a cause-and-effect relationship between insulin and testosterone reporting in a case study the stimulation of ovarian androgen production by insulin, directly correlated to hyperandrogenism (DeClue et al. 1991). On the other hand, insulin promotes the synthesis of DCI (starting from MI) acting directly on the epimerase (Teede, Deeks, and Moran 2010).

Over the years, the critical role of insulin resistance and/or compensatory hyperinsulinemia in the pathogenesis of PCOS have been consistently affirmed throughout the numerous *in vitro* and *in vivo* studies. Indeed, approximately 30–40% of lean women and 80% of obese women with PCOS present the condition of insulin impairment (Baillargeon, Iuorno, and Nestler 2003, Nestler 1997). MI and DCI, both are insulin second messengers and mediate different actions of insulin (Heimark, McAllister, and Larner 2014, Larner et al. 1988). De facto, it was later confirmed that an impairment of the inositol phosphoglycan insulin second messenger pathway might cause a derangement in the insulin signaling in PCOS (Cheang et al. 2008). Hence, the rationale for the use of these two molecules as valuable therapeutic approach of PCOS is designated primarily for their insulin mimetic action (or "insulin sensitizing").

In 1998 an international patent was filed by an International Pharmaceutical Company, INSMED Pharmaceuticals, Inc. (United State patent No. 5.906.979). The inventor of this patent, Professor Geoffrey Allan, President and Director of INSMED Pharmaceuticals, claimed the use of DCI for the treatment of PCOS. These data, based on the use of DCI in the treatment of PCOS patients, published in The New England Journal of Medicine, was considered highly attractive and innovative (Nestler et al. 1999). It was demonstrated that 1200 mg of DCI for 8 weeks could increase insulin sensitivity, improve ovarian function, reduce serum androgens and triglycerides levels in obese patients with PCOS. Ovulation occurred in 86% of these women within 45 days of treatment compared to 27% in the placebo group. INSMED Pharmaceuticals Inc. followed the studies with 600 mg of DCI on lean women with PCOS and the dose-effect was satisfactory (Iuorno et al. 2002). Another study was then designed involving more patients and higher doses of DCI (2400 mg); the results obtained were never published and the launch of the product was discontinued. For confidentiality reasons, the disappointing results were published only in 2008 (Cheang et al. 2008). As a matter of fact, the Scientific Community was surprised to read these discomforting and unexpected results. Particularly, with these higher doses of DCI was not observed an improvement in insulin sensitivity and ovulatory frequency. Could this overdose be the cause of failure? Interestingly, the release of DCI–containing inositol phosphoglycan was not improved in several women after administration of DCI, indicating that these women had a functional aberration in DCI-containing inositol phosphoglycan release, rather than a simple nutritional deficiency of DCI. For the sake of clarity, the lack of efficacy in this study was later correlated to the high dose of DCI.

According to these data, the Insmed Pharmaceutical Company chose to stop completely clinical trials with DCI.

Meanwhile, in 2003, in Italy, the Pharmaceutical Company LO.LI. Pharma concludes the studies on the use of MI in PCOS, obtaining exciting results and a novel Patent (No. 1379164). MI, administered for 6 months twice a day, was effective in restoring spontaneous ovarian activity, and subsequent fertility in PCOS patients (Papaleo et al. 2007). These results were then replicated by other researchers that investigated the metabolic and hormonal effects of MI in PCOS women (Costantino et al. 2009, Genazzani et al. 2008, Gerli et al. 2007, Zacche et al. 2009). An improvement of the hormonal profile and the restoration of ovulation as well as regular menses in both obese and lean women was observed. Up to date, a number of studies have been conducted investigating the effect of inositol on the biochemical and clinical parameters related to hyperandrogenism and metabolism in PCOS women (Artini et al. 2013, Benelli et al. 2016, Colazingari et al. 2013, Genazzani et al. 2008, Gerli, Mignosa, and Di Renzo 2003, Gerli et al. 2007, Nordio and Proietti 2012, Ozay et al. 2016, Pizzo, Lagana, and Barbaro 2014). Collectively all these studies, even with many differences in trial design, sample size, treatment duration and dosage, share a common result: the beneficial effect of MI alone or combined with DCI in improving the metabolic profile of women with PCOS, and a concomitant reduction of hyperandrogenism (Unfer et al. 2017, Unfer et al. 2016).

The Role of Myo-Inositol and D-Chiro-Inositol on Oocyte Quality

In 1992, the role of MI in *in vitro* human fertilization (IVF) was investigated (Chiu and Tam 1992). High level of inositol in the serum samples of patients having successful IVF pregnancies were reported, likely due to its involvement in the early *in vitro* phase of IVF as well as the proper embryonic development. Ten years later, Chiu and collaborators found a correlation between the concentration of MI in the follicular fluid and the quality of the recovered oocytes (i.e., oocytes in meiosis II from mature follicles) (Chiu et al. 2002). Precisely, follicular fluid and serum samples were collected from 53 patients undergoing IVF and statistically analysed for oocyte quality. As a result, the follicles with higher levels of MI contained oocytes of good quality, implying the potential association between MI and inositol phosphates in the phosphatidylinositol cycle activation for oocyte maturation. This gave the prospective of considering the concentration of MI in the follicular fluids as a valuable marker for oocytes of good quality. Few years later, a clinical trial reported the effect of MI in combination with folic acid in inducing spontaneous menstrual cycles and potential pregnancies in PCOS women (Papaleo et al. 2007). The aforementioned findings opened a new scenario and stimulated novel investigations.

The same team, few years later, observed that the amount of recombinant FSH (rFSH) administered and the number of days of stimulation were reduced in those patients with PCOS, undergoing intracytoplasmic sperm injection (ICSI) cycles, treated with MI compared to placebo (Papaleo et al. 2009). The germinal vesicles and degenerated oocytes at ovum pick-up were also reduced after supplementation with MI. Interestingly, in another study, PCOS patients having a normal insulin response, showed an improvement of oocyte and embryo quality during ovarian stimulation protocols after MI treatment rather than DCI (Unfer et al. 2011). This was supposed to be due to the tissue-specific nature of insulin resistance in women with PCOS. In fact, liver and muscle are insulin-resistant in women with PCOS whereas the ovaries retain normal insulin sensitivity (Harwood, Vuguin, and DiMartino-Nardi 2007, Rice et al. 2005). All these findings clearly highlight the beneficial effects on ovarian function and oocyte development, possibly through the action exerted by MI to FSH sensitivity.

The quality of oocytes is a very important factor in the development of a clinical pregnancy, as oocytes of poor quality may lead to infertility and unsuccessful IVF outcomes (Hourvitz et al. 2009). Prior to fertilization the follicular fluid makes up the physical environment for the mature oocyte and may impact IVF outcome parameters like fertilization, embryo cleavage and pregnancy rates. Indeed, during IVF procedures, some morphologically mature oocytes (MII oocytes) from matured follicles might remain unfertilized or yield poor-quality embryo formation (Agarwal, Saleh, and Bedaiwy 2003).

After all these engaging findings, the studies continued enlarging the investigation to molecule combination and different concentrations. In 2010, an Italian team evaluated the efficacy of MI plus melatonin and folic acid on oocyte quality in women undergoing IVF cycles. (Rizzo, Raffone, and Benedetto 2010). As previously observed, melatonin plays a critical role in a number of important physiological functions, having also a direct effect on the female reproductive tract (Nakamura et al. 2003, Woo et al. 2001) and protecting oocytes from oxidative stress (Tamura et al. 2008). The combination of MI plus melatonin and folic acid improved the oocyte quality and pregnancy outcome in women with low oocyte quality history (Rizzo, Raffone, and Benedetto 2010).

Few years later, a total of 54 women with PCOS (maximum age 40 years old) were treated daily for 8 weeks with different concentrations of DCI (300-600-1200-2400 mg) (Isabella and Raffone, 2012). At the end of the study a significant increase in total r-FSH units in the two groups receiving the higher doses of DCI was observed. Furthermore, a significant increase in the number of immature oocytes was seen in the three groups receiving the higher doses of DCI and the number of MII oocytes was significantly lower in the group receiving the highest dosage of DCI compared to placebo group. A reduction of grade I embryos at high DCI levels was reported. De facto, DCI supplementation progressively reduced the oocyte quality and ovarian response.

Recently the correlation with the blastocyst quality and the levels of MI and DCI in follicular fluids in healthy young women was investigated (Ravanos et al. 2017). The blastocysts of good quality correlated with a higher MI/DCI ratio in the follicular fluid, respect to those rated as poor-quality blastocysts. Interestingly, all the transferred blastocysts were graded as good quality, and all of them presented low DCI levels in the follicular fluid. These appealing results showed a clear and significant correlation between MI/DCI ratio in follicular fluid and the blastocyst quality, suggesting that MI/DCI ratio might be a valuable biomarker for blastocysts of good quality, and possible pregnancy success.

THE "DCI PARADOX" IN THE OVARY

Normally, epimerase MI/DCI conversion activity induces a specific MI to DCI ratio that is different in each tissue, but in accordance to its physiological function. Indeed, glycogen storage tissues such as fat, liver and muscle, contain high DCI levels, differently to brain and heart which are tissues with high glucose utilization and contain very low levels of DCI (Larner 2002). Likewise, ovary does not require high doses of DCI for its function. Furthermore, the ratio of these two molecules is insulin dependent as shown in previous studies (Kennington et al. 1990, Sun et al. 2002, Larner and Craig 1996). However, at the systemic level in insulin-resistant and PCOS patients this ratio is altered, due to a decreased epimerase conversion activity (1% vs. 8% in sensitive tissues) and a consequent increase in MI to DCI ratio. On the contrary, in the ovary data showed that epimerase activity is increased, therefore inducing an increase in DCI concentrations and a decrease in MI levels (Bevilacqua et al. 2015). Unlike tissues such as muscle and liver, ovaries never become insulin resistant (Harwood et al. 2007, Matalliotakis et al. 2006, Rice et al. 2005). Carlomagno et al. published a letter reporting that the subsequent depletion of MI might be the cause of poor oocyte quality and the impairment of the FSH signaling (Carlomagno, Unfer, and Roseff 2011). As PCOS women in the ovaries have already high levels of DCI, the supplementation of this molecule would not be the problem-solving approach. At ovarian level it has been shown that MI based second messenger is involved in both glucose uptake and FSH signaling, however DCI-based second messenger is devoted to the insulin-mediated androgen production. According to this, it has been supposed that supplementation of DCI is a valuable treatment for reducing insulin resistance in PCOS patients, but it does not have a beneficial effect at ovarian level (Carlomagno, Unfer, and Roseff 2011).

MI and DCI physiological concentrations in plasma of normal women has been found to be approximately 40:1. This has led researchers to identify the presumably optimal clinical dosage to be transcribed into an effective pharmaceutical treatment. In 2012, the same author Unfer and coll. developed a new pharmaceutical form containing 550 mg of MI and 13.8 mg of DCI (40:1), patented by Lo.Li. Pharma (Carlomagno et al. 2012). In the same year, the synergetic activity of these two molecules was evaluated resulting in an improvement of insulin sensitivity in liver and muscle reducing circulating insulin and restoring FSH sensitivity as well as oocyte quality (Nordio and Proietti 2012).

Furthermore, MI supplementation reduces the rFSH IU administrated during IVF cycles, as observed in previous studies (Larner and Craig 1996, Papaleo et al. 2009, Unfer et al. 2011). This supposedly indicates that the MI depletion in the ovary might be the cause of the FSH signaling impairment, resulting in an increased risk of ovarian hyperstimulation syndrome for PCOS patients.

The so called "DCI paradox" has been widely accepted by the Scientific Community, that reasonably confirmed the effective use of DCI in the treatment of PCOS patients to reduce insulin resistance, however having no effect at ovarian level.

Conclusion

Since the first discovery of inositols in 1850 a lot has been said. The pivotal role, mainly MI and DCI, as a safe and effective treatment of PCOS, has now reached the consensus among scientists and clinicians. Their efficacy in improving oocyte follicular development and oocyte maturation as well as pregnancy outcomes in IVF procedures has been ostensibly recorded. However, the enthusiasm of novel findings and confirmation of existent evidences should and would never stop the research in this field.

REFERENCES

Agarwal, A., R. A. Saleh, and M. A. Bedaiwy. 2003. "Role of reactive oxygen species in the pathophysiology of human reproduction." *Fertil Steril* 79 (4):829-43.

Agranoff, B. W. 2009. "Turtles All the Way: Reflections on myo-Inositol." *J Biol Chem* 284 (32):21121-6. doi: 10.1074/jbc.X109.004747.

Artini, P. G., O. M. Di Berardino, F. Papini, A. D. Genazzani, G. Simi, M. Ruggiero, and V. Cela. 2013. "Endocrine and clinical effects of myo-inositol administration in polycystic ovary syndrome. A randomized study." *Gynecol Endocrinol* 29 (4):375-9. doi: 10.3109/09513590.2012.743020.

Baillargeon, J. P., E. Diamanti-Kandarakis, R. E. Ostlund, Jr., T. Apridonidze, M. J. Iuorno, and J. E. Nestler. 2006. "Altered D-chiro-inositol urinary clearance in women with polycystic ovary syndrome." *Diabetes Care* 29 (2):300-5.

Baillargeon, J. P., M. J. Iuorno, and J. E. Nestler. 2003. "Insulin sensitizers for polycystic ovary syndrome." *Clin Obstet Gynecol* 46 (2):325-40.

Baillargeon, J. P., and J. E. Nestler. 2006. "Commentary: polycystic ovary syndrome: a syndrome of ovarian hypersensitivity to insulin?" *J Clin Endocrinol Metab* 91 (1):22-4. doi: 10.1210/jc.2005-1804.

Barbieri, R. L., A. Makris, R. W. Randall, G. Daniels, R. W. Kistner, and K. J. Ryan. 1986. "Insulin stimulates androgen accumulation in incubations of ovarian stroma obtained from women with hyperandrogenism." *J Clin Endocrinol Metab* 62 (5):904-10. doi: 10.1210/jcem-62-5-904.

Benelli, E., S. Del Ghianda, C. Di Cosmo, and M. Tonacchera. 2016. *A Combined Therapy with Myo-Inositol and D-Chiro-Inositol Improves Endocrine Parameters and Insulin Resistance in PCOS Young Overweight Women*. Vol. 2016.

Bevilacqua, A., G. Carlomagno, S. Gerli, M. Montanino Oliva, P. Devroey, A. Lanzone, C. Soulange, F. Facchinetti, G. Carlo Di Renzo, M. Bizzarri, M. Hod, P. Cavalli, R. D'Anna, S. Benvenga, T. T. Chiu, and Z. A. Kamenov. 2015. "Results from the International Consensus Conference on myo-inositol and D-chiro-inositol in Obstetrics and

Gynecology--assisted reproduction technology." *Gynecol Endocrinol* 31 (6):441-6. doi: 10.3109/09513590.2015.1006616.

Bizzarri, M., A. Fuso, S. Dinicola, A. Cucina, and A. Bevilacqua. 2016. "Pharmacodynamics and pharmacokinetics of inositol(s) in health and disease." *Expert Opin Drug Metab Toxicol* 12 (10):1181-96. doi: 10.1080/17425255.2016.1206887.

Cara, J. F., J. Fan, J. Azzarello, and R. L. Rosenfield. 1990. "Insulin-like growth factor-I enhances luteinizing hormone binding to rat ovarian theca-interstitial cells." *J Clin Invest* 86 (2):560-5. doi: 10.1172/jci114745.

Cara, J. F., and R. L. Rosenfield. 1988. "Insulin-like growth factor I and insulin potentiate luteinizing hormone-induced androgen synthesis by rat ovarian thecal-interstitial cells." *Endocrinology* 123 (2):733-9. doi: 10.1210/endo-123-2-733.

Carlomagno, G., S. De Grazia, V. Unfer, and F. Manna. 2012. "Myo-inositol in a new pharmaceutical form: a step forward to a broader clinical use." *Expert Opin Drug Deliv* 9 (3):267-71. doi: 10.1517/17425247.2012.662953.

Carlomagno, G., V. Unfer, and S. Roseff. 2011. "The D-chiro-inositol paradox in the ovary." *Fertil Steril* 95 (8):2515-6. doi: 10.1016/j.fertnstert.2011.05.027.

Cheang, K. I., J. P. Baillargeon, P. A. Essah, R. E. Ostlund, Jr., T. Apridonize, L. Islam, and J. E. Nestler. 2008. "Insulin-stimulated release of D-chiro-inositol-containing inositolphosphoglycan mediator correlates with insulin sensitivity in women with polycystic ovary syndrome." *Metabolism* 57 (10):1390-7. doi: 10.1016/j.metabol.2008.05.008.

Chiu, T. T., M. S. Rogers, E. L. Law, C. M. Briton-Jones, L. P. Cheung, and C. J. Haines. 2002. "Follicular fluid and serum concentrations of myo-inositol in patients undergoing IVF: relationship with oocyte quality." *Hum Reprod* 17 (6):1591-6.

Chiu, T. T., and P. P. Tam. 1992. "A correlation of the outcome of clinical in vitro fertilization with the inositol content and embryotrophic properties of human serum." *J Assist Reprod Genet* 9 (6):524-30.

Clements, Jr R. S., and B. Darnell. 1980. "Myo-inositol content of common foods: development of a high-myo-inositol diet." *The American Journal of Clinical Nutrition* 33 (9):1954-1967. doi: 10.1093/ajcn/33.9.1954.

Colazingari, S., M. Treglia, R. Najjar, and A. Bevilacqua. 2013. "The combined therapy myo-inositol plus D-chiro-inositol, rather than D-chiro-inositol, is able to improve IVF outcomes: Results from a randomized controlled trial." *Arch Gynecol Obstet.* 288 (6):1405-11. doi: 10.1007/s00404-013-2855-3.

Costantino, D., G. Minozzi, E. Minozzi, and C. Guaraldi. 2009. "Metabolic and hormonal effects of myo-inositol in women with polycystic ovary syndrome: a double-blind trial." *Eur Rev Med Pharmacol Sci* 13 (2):105-10.

de Groot, P. C., O. M. Dekkers, J. A. Romijn, S. W. Dieben, and F. M. Helmerhorst. 2011. "PCOS, coronary heart disease, stroke and the influence of obesity: a systematic review and meta-analysis." *Hum Reprod Update* 17 (4):495-500. doi: 10.1093/humupd/dmr001.

DeClue, T. J., S. C. Shah, M. Marchese, and J. I. Malone. 1991. "Insulin resistance and hyperinsulinemia induce hyperandrogenism in a young type B insulin-resistant female." *J Clin Endocrinol Metab* 72 (6):1308-11. doi: 10.1210/jcem-72-6-1308.

Dunaif, A., Karen Segal, Walter Futterweit, and A. Dobrjansky. 1989. *Profound Peripheral Insulin Resistance, Independent of Obesity, in Polycystic Ovary Syndrome*. Vol. 38.

Dunaif, Andrea. 1997. "Insulin Resistance and the Polycystic Ovary Syndrome: Mechanism and Implications for Pathogenesis*." *Endocrine Reviews* 18 (6):774-800. doi: 10.1210/edrv.18.6.0318.

Ehrmann, D. A., R. B. Barnes, R. L. Rosenfield, M. K. Cavaghan, and J. Imperial. 1999. "Prevalence of impaired glucose tolerance and diabetes in women with polycystic ovary syndrome." *Diabetes Care* 22 (1):141-6.

Eisenberg, F., A. H. Bolden, and F. A. Loewus. 1964. "Inositol formation by cyclization of glucose chain in rat testis." *Biochem Biophys Res Commun* 14:419-24.

Eisenberg, F., Jr., and A. H. Bolden. 1964. "Reproductive tract as site of synthesis and secretion of inositol in the male rat." *Nature* 202:599-600.

Genazzani, A. D., C. Lanzoni, F. Ricchieri, and V. M. Jasonni. 2008. "Myo-inositol administration positively affects hyperinsulinemia and hormonal parameters in overweight patients with polycystic ovary syndrome." *Gynecol Endocrinol* 24 (3):139-44. doi: 10.1080/09513590801893232.

Genazzani, A. D., S. Santagni, F. Ricchieri, A. Campedelli, E. Rattighieri, E. Chierchia, G. Marini, G. Despini, A. Prati, and T. Simoncini. 2014. "Myo-inositol modulates insulin and luteinizing hormone secretion in normal weight patients with polycystic ovary syndrome." *J Obstet Gynaecol Res* 40 (5):1353-60. doi: 10.1111/jog.12319.

Gerli, S., M. Mignosa, and G. C. Di Renzo. 2003. "Effects of inositol on ovarian function and metabolic factors in women with PCOS: a randomized double blind placebo-controlled trial." *Eur Rev Med Pharmacol Sci* 7 (6):151-9.

Gerli, S., E. Papaleo, A. Ferrari, and G. C. Di Renzo. 2007. "Randomized, double blind placebo-controlled trial: effects of myo-inositol on ovarian function and metabolic factors in women with PCOS." *Eur Rev Med Pharmacol Sci* 11 (5):347-54.

Ghafoorunissa. 1976. "Effect of dietary protein & inositol on sperm metabolism & fructose content of male accessory sex organs of rat." *Indian J Exp Biol* 14 (5):564-6.

Hadjiconstantinou, M., H. Mani, N. Patel, M. Levy, M. Davies, K. Khunti, and M. Stone. 2017. "Understanding and supporting women with polycystic ovary syndrome: a qualitative study in an ethnically diverse UK sample." *Endocr Connect* 6 (5):323-330. doi: 10.1530/ec-17-0053.

Harwood, K., P. Vuguin, and J. DiMartino-Nardi. 2007. "Current approaches to the diagnosis and treatment of polycystic ovarian syndrome in youth." *Horm Res* 68 (5):209-17. doi: 10.1159/ 000101538.

Heimark, D., J. McAllister, and J. Larner. 2014. "Decreased myo-inositol to chiro-inositol (M/C) ratios and increased M/C epimerase activity in PCOS theca cells demonstrate increased insulin sensitivity compared to controls." *Endocr J* 61 (2):111-7.

Hourvitz, A., R. Machtinger, E. Maman, M. Baum, J. Dor, and J. Levron. 2009. "Assisted reproduction in women over 40 years of age: how old is too old?" *Reprod Biomed Online* 19 (4):599-603.

Huang, L. C., M. C. Fonteles, D. B. Houston, C. Zhang, and J. Larner. 1993. "Chiroinositol deficiency and insulin resistance. III. Acute glycogenic and hypoglycemic effects of two inositol phosphoglycan insulin mediators in normal and streptozotocin-diabetic rats in vivo." *Endocrinology* 132 (2):652-7. doi: 10.1210/endo.132.2.8425485.

Irvine, R. F. 2016. "A short history of inositol lipids." *Journal of Lipid Research* 57 (11):1987-1994. doi: 10.1194/jlr.R071712.

Isabella, R., and E. Raffone. 2012 "Does ovary need D-chiro-inositol?" *J Ovarian Res* 15 5(1):14.

Iuorno, M. J., D. J. Jakubowicz, J. P. Baillargeon, P. Dillon, R. D. Gunn, G. Allan, and J. E. Nestler. 2002. "Effects of d-chiro-inositol in lean women with the polycystic ovary syndrome." *Endocr Pract* 8 (6):417-23. doi: 10.4158/ep.8.6.417.

Jarrett, J. C., 2nd, G. Ballejo, J. C. Tsibris, and W. N. Spellacy. 1985. "Insulin binding to human ovaries." *J Clin Endocrinol Metab* 60 (3):460-3. doi: 10.1210/jcem-60-3-460.

Kennington, A. S., C. R. Hill, J. Craig, C. Bogardus, I. Raz, H. K. Ortmeyer, B. C. Hansen, G. Romero, and J. Larner. 1990. "Low Urinary chiro-Inositol Excretion in Non-Insulin-Dependent Diabetes Mellitus." *New England Journal of Medicine* 323 (6):373-378. doi: 10.1056/NEJM199008093230603.

Larner, J. 2002. "D-chiro-inositol--its functional role in insulin action and its deficit in insulin resistance." *Int J Exp Diabetes Res* 3 (1):47-60.

Larner, J., L. C. Huang, G. Tang, S. Suzuki, C. F. Schwartz, G. Romero, Z. Roulidis, K. Zeller, T. Y. Shen, A. S. Oswald, and et al. 1988. "Insulin mediators: structure and formation." *Cold Spring Harb Symp Quant Biol* 53 Pt 2:965-71.

Larner, J., and J. W. Craig. 1996. "Urinary myo-inositol-to-chiro-inositol ratios and insulin resistance." *Diabetes Care* 19 (1):76.

Legro, R. S., A. R. Kunselman, W. C. Dodson, and A. Dunaif. 1999. "Prevalence and Predictors of Risk for Type 2 Diabetes Mellitus and

Impaired Glucose Tolerance in Polycystic Ovary Syndrome: A Prospective, Controlled Study in 254 Affected Women." *The Journal of Clinical Endocrinology & Metabolism* 84 (1):165-169. doi: 10.1210/jcem.84.1.5393.

Lewin, L. M., and R. Beer. 1973. "Prostatic secretion as the source of myo-inositol in human seminal fluid." *Fertil Steril* 24 (9):666-70.

Lim, S. S., M. J. Davies, R. J. Norman, and L. J. Moran. 2012. "Overweight, obesity and central obesity in women with polycystic ovary syndrome: a systematic review and meta-analysis." *Hum Reprod Update* 18 (6):618-37. doi: 10.1093/humupd/dms030.

Majumder, A. L., and B. B. Biswas. 2006. *Biology of Inositols and Phosphoinositides*, *Subcellular Biochemistry*: Springer US.

Maquenne, L.. 1887a. "Préparation, proprietés et constitution se l'inosite." *Comptes Rendus Hebdomadaires Des Seances De l'Academie Des Sciences* ["Preparation, proprieties and constitution is inosite." *Weekly Reports of Sessions of the Academy of Sciences*] 104:225-227.

Maquenne, L.. 1887b. "Sur les propriétés de l'inosite." *Comptes rendus hebdomadaires des séances de l'Académie des sciences* 104:297-299.

Maquenne, L.. 1887c. "Sur quelques dérivés de l'inosite." *Comptes Rendus Hebdomadaires Des Seances De l'Academie Des Sciences* 104:1719-1722.

Matalliotakis, I., A. Kourtis, O. Koukoura, D. Panidis. 2006. "Polycystic ovary syndrome: etiology and pathogenesis." *Arch Gynecol Obstet* 274: 187–97.

Murthy, P. P. 2006. "Structure and nomenclature of inositol phosphates, phosphoinositides, and glycosylphosphatidylinositols." *Subcell Biochem* 39:1-19.

Nakamura, Y., H. Tamura, H. Takayama, and H. Kato. 2003. "Increased endogenous level of melatonin in preovulatory human follicles does not directly influence progesterone production." *Fertil Steril* 80 (4):1012-6.

Nestler, J. E. 1997. "Role of hyperinsulinemia in the pathogenesis of the polycystic ovary syndrome, and its clinical implications." *Semin Reprod Endocrinol* 15 (2):111-22. doi: 10.1055/s-2007-1016294.

Nestler, J. E., D. J. Jakubowicz, P. Reamer, R. D. Gunn, and G. Allan. 1999. "Ovulatory and metabolic effects of D-chiro-inositol in the polycystic ovary syndrome." *N Engl J Med* 340 (17):1314-20. doi: 10.1056/nejm199904293401703.

Nordio, M., and E. Proietti. 2012. "The combined therapy with myo-inositol and D-chiro-inositol reduces the risk of metabolic disease in PCOS overweight patients compared to myo-inositol supplementation alone." *Eur Rev Med Pharmacol Sci* 16 (5):575-81.

Ozay, A., O. E. Ozay, R. E. Okyay, E. Cagliyan, T. Küme, and B. Gulekli. 2016. *Different Effects of Myoinositol plus Folic Acid versus Combined Oral Treatment on Androgen Levels in PCOS Women*. Vol. 2016.

Pak, Y., L. C. Huang, K. J. Lilley, and J. Larner. 1992. "In vivo conversion of [3H]myoinositol to [3H]chiroinositol in rat tissues." *J Biol Chem* 267 (24):16904-10.

Palomba, S., S. Santagni, A. Falbo, and G. B. La Sala. 2015. "Complications and challenges associated with polycystic ovary syndrome: current perspectives." *Int J Womens Health* 7:745-63. doi: 10.2147/ijwh.s70314.

Papaleo, E., V. Unfer, J. P. Baillargeon, L. De Santis, F. Fusi, C. Brigante, G. Marelli, I. Cino, A. Redaelli, and A. Ferrari. 2007. "Myo-inositol in patients with polycystic ovary syndrome: a novel method for ovulation induction." *Gynecol Endocrinol* 23 (12):700-3. doi: 10.1080/09513590701672405.

Papaleo, E., V. Unfer, J. P. Baillargeon, F. Fusi, F. Occhi, and L. De Santis. 2009. "Myo-inositol may improve oocyte quality in intracytoplasmic sperm injection cycles. A prospective, controlled, randomized trial." *Fertil Steril* 91 (5):1750-4. doi: 10.1016/j. fertnstert.2008.01.088.

Pizzo, A., A. S. Lagana, and L. Barbaro. 2014. "Comparison between effects of myo-inositol and D-chiro-inositol on ovarian function and metabolic factors in women with PCOS." *Gynecol Endocrinol* 30 (3):205-8. doi: 10.3109/09513590.2013.860120.

Poretsky, L., F. Grigorescu, M. Seibel, A. C. Moses, and J. S. Flier. 1985. "Distribution and characterization of insulin and insulin-like growth factor I receptors in normal human ovary." *J Clin Endocrinol Metab* 61 (4):728-34. doi: 10.1210/jcem-61-4-728.

Poretsky, L., D. Smith, M. Seibel, A. Pazianos, A. C. Moses, and J. S. Flier. 1984. "Specific insulin binding sites in human ovary." *J Clin Endocrinol Metab* 59 (4):809-11. doi: 10.1210/jcem-59-4-809.

Qin, J. Z., L. H. Pang, M. J. Li, X. J. Fan, R. D. Huang, and H. Y. Chen. 2013. "Obstetric complications in women with polycystic ovary syndrome: a systematic review and meta-analysis." *Reprod Biol Endocrinol* 11:56. doi: 10.1186/1477-7827-11-56.

Ravanos, K., G. Monastra, T. Pavlidou, M. Goudakou, and N. Prapas. 2017. "Can high levels of D-chiro-inositol in follicular fluid exert detrimental effects on blastocyst quality?" *Eur Rev Med Pharmacol Sci.* 21 (23):5491-5498. doi: 10.26355/eurrev_201712_13940.

Rice, S., N. Christoforidis, C. Gadd, D. Nikolaou, L. Seyani, A. Donaldson, R. Margara, K. Hardy, and S. Franks. 2005. "Impaired insulin-dependent glucose metabolism in granulosa-lutein cells from anovulatory women with polycystic ovaries." *Hum Reprod* 20 (2):373-81. doi: 10.1093/humrep/deh609.

Rizzo, M., K. Berneis, G. Spinas, G. B. Rini, and E. Carmina. 2009. "Long-term consequences of polycystic ovary syndrome on cardiovascular risk." *Fertil Steril* 91 (4 Suppl):1563-7. doi: 10.1016/j.fertnstert.2008.09.070.

Rizzo, P., E. Raffone, and V. Benedetto. 2010. "Effect of the treatment with myo-inositol plus folic acid plus melatonin in comparison with a treatment with myo-inositol plus folic acid on oocyte quality and pregnancy outcome in IVF cycles. A prospective, clinical trial." *Eur Rev Med Pharmacol Sci* 14 (6):555-61.

Scherer, Johann Joseph. 1850. "Uber eine neue aus dem Muskelfleisch gewonnene Zuckerart." *Liebigs Annalen der Chemie* 73:322.

Spector, R., and A. V. Lorenzo. 1975a. "Myo-inositol transport in the central nervous system." *Am J Physiol* 228 (5):1510-18. doi: 10.1152/ajplegacy.1975.228.5.1510.

Spector, R., and A. V. Lorenzo. 1975b. "The origin of myo-inositol in brain, cerebrospinal fluid and choroid plexus." *J Neurochem* 25 (3):353-4.

Stein, I. F., and M. L. Leventhal. 1935. "Amenorrhea associated with bilateral polycystic ovaries." *American Journal of Obstetrics & Gynecology* 29 (2):181-191. doi: 10.1016/S0002-9378(15)30642-6.

Sun, T. H., D. B. Heimark, T. Nguygen, J. L. Nadler, and J. Larner. 2002. "Both myo-inositol to chiro-inositol epimerase activities and chiro-inositol to myo-inositol ratios are decreased in tissues of GK type 2 diabetic rats compared to Wistar controls." *Biochem Biophys Res Commun* 293 (3):1092-8. doi: 10.1016/s0006-291x(02)00313-3.

Tamura, H., A. Takasaki, I. Miwa, K. Taniguchi, R. Maekawa, H. Asada, T. Taketani, A. Matsuoka, Y. Yamagata, K. Shimamura, H. Morioka, H. Ishikawa, R. J. Reiter, and N. Sugino. 2008. "Oxidative stress impairs oocyte quality and melatonin protects oocytes from free radical damage and improves fertilization rate." *J Pineal Res* 44 (3):280-7. doi: 10.1111/j.1600-079X.2007.00524.x.

Teede, H., A. Deeks, and L. Moran. 2010. "Polycystic ovary syndrome: a complex condition with psychological, reproductive and metabolic manifestations that impacts on health across the lifespan." *BMC Med* 8:41. doi: 10.1186/1741-7015-8-41.

Unfer, V., G. Carlomagno, P. Rizzo, E. Raffone, and S. Roseff. 2011. "Myo-inositol rather than D-chiro-inositol is able to improve oocyte quality in intracytoplasmic sperm injection cycles. A prospective, controlled, randomized trial." *Eur Rev Med Pharmacol Sci* 15 (4):452-7.

Unfer, V., F. Facchinetti, B. Orrù, B. Giordani, and J. Nestler. 2017. "Myo-inositol effects in women with PCOS: a meta-analysis of randomized controlled trials." *Endocr Connect* 6 (8):647-658. doi: 10.1530/ec-17-0243.

Unfer, V., J. E. Nestler, Z. A. Kamenov, N. Prapas, and F. Facchinetti. 2016. "Effects of Inositol(s) in Women with PCOS: A Systematic Review of Randomized Controlled Trials." *International Journal of Endocrinology* 2016:12. doi: 10.1155/2016/1849162.

Voglmayr, J. K., and R. P. Amann. 1973. "The Distribution of Free Myo-Inositol in Fluids, Spermatozoa, and Tissues of the Bull Genital Tract and Observations on its Uptake by the Rabbit Epididymis." *Biology of Reproduction* 8 (4):504-513. doi: 10.1093/biolreprod/8.4.504.

Wang, W. T., J. Safar, and D. Zopf. 1990. "Analysis of inositol by high-performance liquid chromatography." *Anal Biochem* 188 (2):432-5.

Woo, M. M., C. J. Tai, S. K. Kang, P. S. Nathwani, S. F. Pang, and P. C. Leung. 2001. "Direct action of melatonin in human granulosa-luteal cells." *J Clin Endocrinol Metab* 86 (10):4789-97. doi: 10.1210/jcem.86.10.7912.

Zacche, M. M., L. Caputo, S. Filippis, G. Zacche, M. Dindelli, and A. Ferrari. 2009. "Efficacy of myo-inositol in the treatment of cutaneous disorders in young women with polycystic ovary syndrome." *Gynecol Endocrinol* 25 (8):508-13. doi: 10.1080/09513590903015544.

In: Inositols
Editor: Vittorio Unfer
ISBN: 978-1-53614-912-8

Chapter 2

EATING EXTRA DIETARY INOSITOL: HOW DOES IT COUNTER THE IMPACTS OF METABOLIC, NUTRITIONAL AND ENDOCRINE IMBALANCES?

Robert H. Michell*, PhD

School of Biosciences, University of Birmingham,
Birmingham, UK

ABSTRACT

Myo-inositol (Ins) is a cyclic polyol (hexahydroxy*cyclo*hexane) that is an essential component of the headgroups of some of the membrane phospholipids of eukaryote cells. Ins is a necessary but fairly abundant nutrient, and by the 1980s it was widely assumed that a combination of diet and endogenous synthesis gives us an adequate Ins supply, so studies of dietary Ins deficiency dwindled. However, a few accounts continued to suggest that extra Ins might alleviate some diabetic and teratological pathologies, and a body of evidence has since accumulated which suggests

* Corresponding Author's Email: r.h.michell@bham.ac.uk.

that substantial Ins supplements alleviate some metabolic and endocrine human maladies (including the obstetric and gynaecological conditions discussed in this book) and several types of experimentally induced fatty livers. These all tend to display overlapping constellations of metabolic and endocrine imbalances that include obesity/overweight, non-alcoholic fatty liver disease (NAFLD), tissue insulin resistance, hyperinsulinaemia, and endoplasmic reticulum (ER) stress in the affected tissues. Despite the recognition of this pattern, we still do not know why taking extra Ins helps in these conditions. Tissues probably use most of the extra Ins to make phosphatidylinositol (PtdIns), which is by far the most abundant inositol phospholipid, and PtdIns will in most cells be mainly in the ER, which is usually the largest membrane system. I recently suggested the following as a unifying explanation of the benefits of Ins supplements: ER stress is a common feature of the Ins-responsive conditions; remediation of ER stress requires assembly of more ER membrane by biosynthetic processes that must supply 'extra' PtdIns (and other ER membrane phospholipids); supplementing the Ins supply lets mildly Ins-depleted tissues make more PtdIns; and the resulting ER expansion speeds the restoration of normal ER functions, allowing the resolution of other tissue imbalances (Michell 2018). Here I discuss some of the evidence germane to this interpretation.

Keywords: insulin resistance, NAFLD, lipid droplets, phosphoinositides, phosphatidylinositol, endoplasmic reticulum stress

INTRODUCTION

Eukaryotic and Archaeal Cell Membranes Contain Phospholipids with a D-*myo-inositol* 1-Phosphate (Ins1*P*) Headgroup

Until the mid-20th century, *myo-inositol* (Ins) was mainly known as a chemically stable sugar-like substance that is widely distributed in plants and animals. It was known to be a necessary nutrient for eukaryotic organisms and/or for cells that cannot make any or enough Ins – including some yeasts and many cells in tissue culture. Dietary Ins was beneficial for animals fed Ins-depleted diets, especially if they were lactating or were over-fed with saturated fat, and also for animals faced with some liver-targeted metabolic stresses such as choline deficiency (Holub 1986, Kuksis and Mookerjea 1978, Wells 1989).

Ins-containing membrane phospholipids, known collectively as phosphoinositides, have headgroups based on D-*myo-inositol* 1-phosphate (Ins1*P*). In the mid-20th century they were found in a few phylogenetically scattered organisms: animals, plants, fungi and some bacteria (Hawthorne 1960).

Although Ins1*P*-based phosphoinositides were first discovered in actinobacteria, we have since realised that relatively few bacteria contain and/or make them. By contrast, genomic and biochemical studies suggest that most of the Archaea – the non-bacterial domain of prokaryotic micro-organisms from which many workers believe that some of the extra-mitochondrial Biology of eukaryote cells evolved (Williams and Embley 2015) – synthesize Ins3*P* from glucose 6-phosphate, and that most archaeal cell membranes contain Ins1*P*-based phospholipids (Michell 2008, Morii et al. 2014). Much of the little we know about phosphoinositides in Archaea has come from genomic inferences rather than direct cell-biological, biochemical or metabolic observations. When we get more information on the Biology of archaeal phosphoinositides it should offer valuable hints as to why phosphoinositides have been retained as essential eukaryotic membrane constituents ever since the evolutionary transition that functionally integrated cellular elements of certain early archaea into the Last Eukaryotic Common Ancestor (LECA) from which all other eukaryotes are descended.

There have been hints, as yet unconfirmed, that some cells might contain small amounts of phospholipids with inositol isomers other than Ins in their headgroups (e.g., *scyllo*-inositol; Ryals and Kersting 1999: D-*chiro*-inositol; Pak et al. 1993).

Eight eukaryotic phosphoinositides, with Ins1*P* headgroups that are either unadorned or modified by one, two or three more phosphate groups, have many functions. During the last half century or so, studies of diverse eukaryotic organisms and cells have led to a remarkable understanding of the complex array of roles that these phosphoinositides play in the cells of all eukaryotes (Choy, Han, and Botelho 2017, Di Paolo and De Camilli 2006, Fruman et al. 2017, Irvine 2016, Michell 2008, 2018, Wallroth and Haucke 2017). As a result, an encyclopaedic review by Balla (2013) was justifiably entitled "Phosphoinositides: tiny lipids with giant impact on cell regulation."

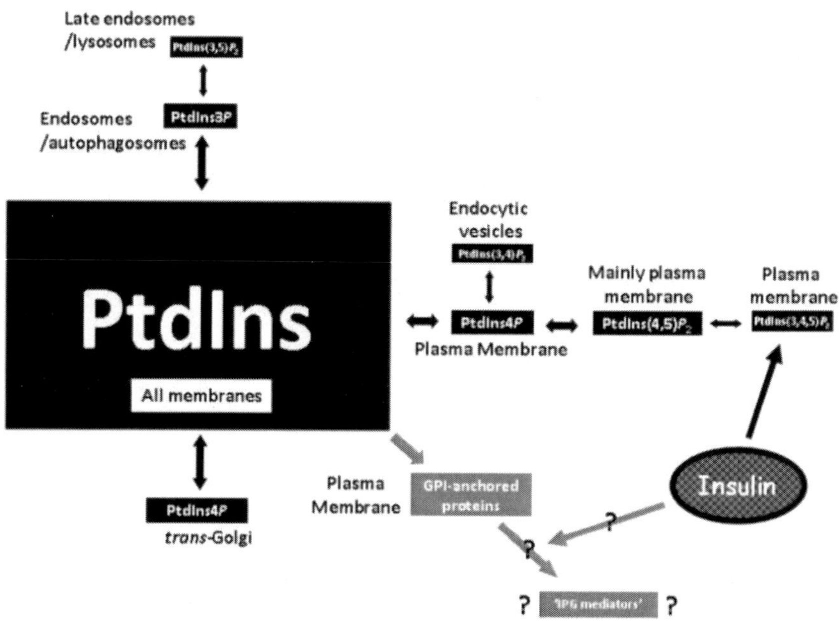

Figure 1. A schematic depiction of: a) the relative quantities in a 'typical' mammalian cell of PtdIns and of the various PPIn with which it continuously inter-converted; and b) established and postulated roles of phosphoinositide derivatives in insulin signalling (bottom right). The sizes of the text-boxes give a very approximate representation of the relative abundances of the named phosphoinositides, and the text alongside each PPIn identifies predominant cellular site(s) at which it is found (for more detailed information, see Balla, 2014; Choy, Han and Botelho, 2017; Wallroth and Haucke, 2018). PtdIns4*P* appears twice because PtdIns4*P* pools made by different PtdIns 4-kinases fulfil very different functions at the plasma membrane and the *trans*-Golgi. PtdIns5*P* is omitted because its very low abundance would make it unreadable at any likely scale of reproduction. Discussion of the relative roles in insulin signalling of PtdIns(3,4,5)P_3 and of 'IPGs' (at bottom right) appears later in the text.

Many of these discoveries can be summarised thus (for further information see also the reviews listed above):

- Eukaryotic cells make quite a lot of phosphatidylinositol (*sn*-1,2-diacylglycero-3-phospho-D-1-*myo-inositol*, abbreviated as PtdIns) – or occasionally other closely related diradylGro3*P*1Ins-based lipid(s) such as those in *Dictyostelium* (Clark et al. 2014).
- PtdIns is made at the cytoplasmic face of the endoplasmic reticulum (ER) from phosphatidate (PtdOH) by a two-step pathway that is catalysed by integral ER membrane enzymes: CDP-diacylglycerol synthases (encoded by CDS1 and CDS2) convert PtdOH to CDP-diacylglycerol (CDP-DG), and this serves as the phosphatidyl donor for PtdIns formation by PtdIns synthase (PIS) (Bochud and Conzelmann 2015).
- ER-synthesised PtdIns is then distributed amongst the cytosol-facing lipid leaflets of all of the membranes of the cell (maybe except the inner mitochondrial membrane) (see Figure 1). This process is catalysed at least in part by phospholipid exchange proteins that act at contact zones between the ER and other cell membranes (Balla 2013, Cockcroft and Raghu 2018, Kim, Hernandez, and Balla 2013, Stefan et al. 2017, Wong, Čopič, and Levine 2017).
- Phosphoinositides usually constitute ~5-20% of the phospholipids of eukaryote cells.
- Most of the PtdIns in the ER remains unmodified; but various proportions of the cytosol-exposed PtdIns in a cell's other membrane systems are rapidly inter-converted (by kinase/phosphatase cycles) between PtdIns and 3- and/or 4- and/or 5-phosphorylated PtdIns derivatives (Figure 1). These seven **P**oly**P**hospho**In**ositides are collectively abbreviated as PPIn.
- Each of the PPIn is made and functions in one or more defined cellular membrane compartments, where it fulfils specific functions. We do not yet know with any accuracy how much of the PtdIns in each of the cell's organelle systems exists at any moment as PtdIns

or as each of the various PPIn – or how rapidly these are interconverted (Choy, Han, and Botelho 2017, Wallroth and Haucke 2017).

- Examples of the compartment-specific functions of PPIn include: PtdIns(4,5)P_2 is mainly in the plasma membrane (PM), where it is the substrate for two transmembrane signalling pathways and is implicated, *inter alia*, in regulating cell motility, exocytosis, ciliary protein delivery and some ion channels; PtdIns3P is essential for correct membrane trafficking through endosomal and autophagosomal compartments; and PtdIns(3,5)P_2 is localised in the membranes of acidified endolysosomal compartments wherein it regulates diverse processes, including membrane trafficking and the activities of some ion channels (Dove et al. 2009, Ho, Alghamdi, and Botelho 2012; and see Figure 1).
- The many PPIn-selective functions are executed by effector proteins that employ various types of PPIn-binding protein domains (PH, FYVE, Tubby, PX, etc.) to become correctly localised to and to function in response to the headgroups of particular PPIn. Some of the PPIn effector proteins also interact with a second partner protein, in a process known as 'coincidence detection', and this extra binding affinity and protein selectivity adds further refinement to the spatial targeting of their intracellular actions (Hammond and Balla 2015, Lemmon 2008).
- A small amount of the PtdIns in the ER is trafficked to the luminal face of the membrane, thence to undergo a complex set of transformations and translocations – as a result of which it is incorporated into the 'glycosylphosphatidylinositol (GPI) anchors' that moor many proteins into the outer leaflet of the PM (Zurzolo and Simons 2016).
- Eukaryotic cells also contain diverse water-soluble Ins polyphosphates, many of which are direct or indirect metabolic products of the Ins(1,4,5)P_3 liberated by the phosphoinositidase C signalling pathway. I will not consider these further.

The ER Usually Contains Much of the Cell's Abundant PtdIns

Eukaryote cells of various types contain quite a lot of PtdIns and much smaller amounts of various PPIn (Figure 1), with their PPIn complements ranging from just two types (PtdIns4*P* and PtdIns(4,5)P_2) in mature mammalian erythrocytes that only have a plasma membrane to at least seven types (PtdIns3*P*, PtdIns4*P*, PtdIns5*P*, PtdIns(3,4)P_2, PtdIns(4,5)P_2, PtdIns(3,5)P_2 and PtdIns(3,4,5)P_3) in complex metazoan tissue cells that employ various PPIn for multiple signalling, membrane trafficking and other functions.

The ER is the most extensive membrane system in many eukaryote cells, and much (or most?) of a cell's unmodified PtdIns resides there. By contrast, each of the much rarer PPIn tends to be localised to one (or a subset) of the cell's less abundant and non-mitochondrial membrane compartments – the PM and its sub-domains, clathrin-coated endocytic vesicles, the Golgi complex and its sub-compartments, late endosomes, autophagosomes, lysosomes/vacuoles, etc. (see Figure 1; Choy, Han, and Botelho 2017, Hammond and Balla 2015, Wallroth and Haucke 2017).

Our current understanding of the diverse functions of PPIn has been brought about largely as a result of the ingenuity with which workers in many laboratories have devised fluorescence labelling and enzymatic tools that can be expressed in localised and tightly regulated ways within living cells. By using these, it is possible to monitor where in the cells the various PPIn are and the temporal changes in their concentrations, experimentally to increase or decrease their local intracellular concentrations, and to determine the effects of these changes on specific cell functions (Choy, Han, and Botelho 2017, Di Paolo and De Camilli 2006, Hammond and Balla 2015, Idevall-Hagren and De Camilli 2015, Wallroth and Haucke 2017).

However, it is easy to forget: a) that the currently available techniques only monitor, and not always with precise fidelity, the changes in local abundance and functions of various PPIn; b) that each of the PPIn is a rare PtdIns derivative; c) and that *in most cells the total cellular PPIn complement represents no more than a few percent of a cell's phosphoinositides* – but that a single PPIn might occasionally dominate the membranes of a small organelle compartment or of a sub-domain therein.

Most of a cell's phosphoinositide is the much more abundant PtdIns, and much of it is in the extensive and largely PPIn-free ER membrane system – *and PtdIns is invisible to the analytical techniques just mentioned.* In the lipid bilayer of the ER membrane PtdIns is mixed with much larger quantities of phosphatidylcholine (PtdCho) and phosphatidylethanolamine (PtdEtn), with a little phosphatidylserine (PtdSer) and cholesterol, and probably only with transient traces of PPIn (mainly short-lived PtdIns4*P*, whenever this exchanges in from other membranes; and PtdIns3*P* that is made at ER-associated autophagic initiation sites) (Choy, Han, and Botelho 2017, English and Voeltz 2013, Holthuis and Menon 2014, Joshi, Zhang, and Prinz 2017, Nishimura et al. 2017).

Dietary Ins Requirements of Mammals, and Possible Benefits of Dietary Ins Supplementation

Evidence on this question has accumulated in several phases since the mid-20th century (see below). Initially there were formal studies of the effects of Ins deficiency in animal models, and especially of the ability of Ins feeding to ameliorate the development of fatty livers in Ins-deficient animals. A second set of information, accumulated during recent decades, has suggested that feeding extra Ins to people afflicted by various metabolic/endocrine diseases (or to animal models thereof) may reduce the severity of some of the clinical manifestations of these conditions. And, finally, recent reports of genetic interventions in the synthesis and cellular distribution of PtdIns have reported effects that are reminiscent of events seen in the historic Ins deficiency studies.

The early work on dietary Ins restriction and supplementation in mammals established that it is quite difficult to provoke an overt Ins deficiency syndrome in healthy and well-fed laboratory rodents. To reveal such a deficiency usually requires *both* the removal of Ins from the diet *and* some coexisting metabolic or genetic stressor such as lactation, high fat feeding, drug-induced diabetes mellitus or antibiotic ablation of Ins-synthesising gut flora (Wells 1989). The commonest Ins-reversible tissue pathologies seen during Ins deficiency were hair loss (Woolley 1941) and accumulations of intracellular fat in the liver and/or in the intestinal mucosa (Holub 1986, Kuksis and Mookerjea 1978, Wells 1989).

Extra Ins intake ameliorates the hepatic effects of these Ins deficiencies, and it can also help to resolve fatty livers that are provoked by a growing variety of treatments other than deliberate Ins deprivation. Examples, listed in Table 1, include: protein starvation, choline deficiency, a very high fat diet, high sucrose or high fructose diets, intraperitoneal administration of Triton WR-1339 and exposure to the hepatotoxic chlorinated insecticide DDT (1,1,1-trichloro-2,2-*bis*(*p*-chlorophenyl)ethane). And there is even a very early report that preoperative Ins administration to human patients undergoing gastrointestinal cancer surgery may ameliorate their fatty livers (Abels et al. 1943).

Table 1. Fatty liver/NAFLD/TAFLD conditions that resolve, at least in part, following dietary Ins supplementation

Stresses that give rise to fatty liver/NAFLD	**References** Detailed discussions of early studies can be found in Holub (1976) and Wells (1989).
Gastrointestinal cancers	Abels et al. 1943.
Ins deficiency	Hayashi, Maeda and Tomita, 1974; Hayashi et al. 1978.
Protein starvation	Macfarland and McHenry, 1948.
Choline deficiency	Kotaki et al. 1968; Yagi and Kotaki, 1969.
High saturated fat diet	Anderson and Holub, 1976; Croze, Géloën and Soulage 2015.
High sucrose/fructose diet	Katayama, 1997, 1999; Shimada, Hibino and Takeshita, 2017.
Intraperitoneal Triton WR-1339 administration	Antony et al. 2017
Toxic challenge with DDT	Okazaki and Katayama, 2003; Okazaki, Setoguchi and Katayama 2006.
Lactation	Burton and Wells, 1976.

By the 1980s it seemed likely that one important reason for the Ins-responsiveness of the intracellular fat accumulations in tissues affected by overt Ins deficiency is that re-supplying Ins corrects a partial failure in Ins-deficient animals of the secretion into the bloodstream of ApoB-containing lipoproteins: VLDL from liver and/or chylomicra from intestinal mucosa (Abels et al. 1943, Nishigaki et al. 1971, Wells 1989). An apparently alternative opinion (but see later) was that adipose tissue lipolysis in the Ins-deficient animals liberates fatty acids that are harvested into the fat-overloaded liver (Hayashi et al. 1978, Hayashi, Maeda, and Tomita 1974). However, by that period it was becoming accepted that a combination of an average mixed diet and endogenous Ins3*P* biosynthesis usually supplies enough Ins for health (Clements Jr and Darnell 1980), so most researchers simply stopped studying Ins deficiency.

More recently, it has become increasingly apparent that at least some people who are afflicted by various metabolic/endocrine diseases obtain benefit – for still unknown reasons – if they eat a few grams of extra Ins a day. The responsive conditions are briefly summarised in Table 1 of Michell (2018), where additional references can be found.

It has been known for quite some time that supplementary Ins is helpful: a) in reducing the number of diabetes-induced birth defects and large-for-gestational age babies born to diabetic pregnant women (Beemster, Groenen and Steegers-Theunissen 2002, Greene, Leung and Copp 2017); b) for reducing the frequency of neural tube defects in genetically susceptible *curly tail* mice (Greene and Copp 1997, Greene, Leung, and Copp 2017); and c) for reducing the risks of compromised lung function and retinopathy in premature babies (Hallman 2015). Several other common conditions, and their associated risks, have since been found to respond positively – at least in some patients – to the taking of Ins supplements (for detailed information, see Croze and Soulage 2013, Dinicola et al. 2017, Michell 2018; and other chapters in this book). These include:

- improved hormone balance, more regular menstruation and ovulation, and better fertility outcomes in women with polycystic ovarian syndrome (PCOS);

- decreased incidence of metabolic syndrome and gestational diabetes in young women;
- some evidence of improved insulin sensitivity and glucose handling in patients with metabolic syndrome or Type II diabetes;
- improved sperm quality in some sub-fertile men; and
- improved *in vitro* embryo development in Ins-containing media, leading to better pregnancy outcomes during assisted conception procedures.

Thirdly, a few recent studies of the genetic depletion or ablation of enzymes needed for PtdIns synthesis or of exchange proteins that may be involved in PtdIns distribution around cells have refocused attention on hepatic and other steatoses that are caused, at least in part, by some combination of the lipid accumulation and/or slowed lipoprotein export that occur when cells cannot be sure of an adequate PtdIns supply (Alb et al. 2007, Liu et al. 2014, Michell 2018, Thakur et al. 2013, Thakur et al. 2011).

How Might Ins Supplements Bring Benefits in Metabolic Diseases and During Nutritional Challenges?

What do these clinical and experimental observations have in common, and how does eating extra Ins confer advantage on a variety of different tissues in such apparently diverse situations? It seems fairly certain that they all involve some degree of mild functional Ins deficiency that can be corrected by eating more Ins. The Ins-responsive patients and animals had been keeping going without obvious problems until: a) their systems were faced with an increased intensity of 'normal' metabolic demands, such as those imposed by pregnancy or lactation; or b) they were afflicted by one of the clinical conditions just listed; or c) they were nutritionally overloaded, often by an obesogenic diet rich in saturated fat and/or fructose-rich carbohydrate; or d) they were assailed by a hepatotoxic stress such as DDT; or e) they encountered some combination of the above.

It seems likely that such stresses unmask the covert consequences of a pre-existing, but subclinical, Ins deficit that is corrected by eating extra Ins. This type of metabolic pattern has been well documented in diabetes mellitus and polycystic ovarian syndrome (PCOS) (Croze and Soulage 2013, Dinicola et al. 2017, Michell 2018), but it is by no means established that this type of hidden, but functionally important, Ins deficit is a common feature of the other conditions.

The remainder of this discussion will briefly consider how such a mild Ins deficiency might come about and how alleviating it could be beneficial. It will make the simplifying assumption, which has been justified elsewhere (Michell 2018), that we should try to identify and understand a single basic PtdIns-dependent mechanism that goes awry in a manner that can be corrected by alleviating a mild Ins deficit.

How Do These Mild Ins Deficiency States Come About?

Two key ideas about ways in which Ins might be lost from the body, precipitating a mild Ins deficiency, have flowed from studies of human diabetes and of animal models of diabetes. First, hyperglycaemia and glycosuria suppress renal tubular re-absorption of filtered Ins by the kidney, facilitating Ins loss in the urine. This has been recognised for more than half a century (Daughaday, Larner, and Houghton 1954, Hong et al. 2012, Kawa, Przybylski, and Taylor 2003, Larner, Brautigan, and Thorner 2010, Murphy et al. 2016). Secondly, high blood glucose, hyperinsulinaemia and high fat feeding all stimulate the activity of renal tubular myo-inositol oxidase (MIOX), the enzyme responsible for the body's only direct catabolic route of Ins loss (Croze and Soulage 2013, Dinicola et al. 2017, Michell 2018, Nayak et al. 2011, Tominaga et al. 2015). Moreover, there is evidence that some polymorphisms of the MIOX gene somehow influence the likelihood that individuals will develop diabetes (Yang et al. 2010).

A third possible contributor to the development of a mild Ins deficiency, discussed by Schlemmer et al. (2009), Dinicola et al. (2017), and Duong, Lapsley, and Pegg (2018), is that the preparation processes for some modern foods might sometimes influence the quantity and availability of dietary Ins, leading to unregulated variations of Ins intake within and between human populations. The assessment of dietary Ins intake – as free Ins liberated from digested foods, as intact diet-derived InsP_6 (phytate), or in both forms – has until recently been confused by inadequately validated studies of the alleged intestinal absorption, systemic circulation and urinary excretion of intact InsP_6. And some of these observations have been offered in support of the questionable idea that intact extracellular InsP_6 might have important anti-cancer effects (Vucenik and Shamsuddin 2006).

It always seemed unlikely that intact InsP_6, which is a very charge-dense polyanion, would be absorbed from gut contents through intestinal mucosal membranes, and this notion now seems to have been invalidated by careful studies that: a) found no detectable InsP_6 in human blood plasma or urine; and b) found an InsP_6 phosphatase (phytase) activity in human plasma that would quickly degrade any InsP_6 that did get into the bloodstream (Irvine et al. 2015). It therefore seems fairly certain – irrespective of what combined forms of Ins we eat and of what local effects ingested InsP_6 might have within the gut lumen – that the dietary Ins that we absorb, that circulates and that is delivered to our tissues will be free Ins.

Correcting an Ins Deficit Reverts the Sensitivity of Insulin-Resistant Tissues towards Normal

Some or all of a constellation of coexisting features/symptoms are shared by several of the Ins-responsive human conditions (including PCOS, metabolic syndrome, gestational diabetes and Type II diabetes) and by animal models of obesity, of diabetes and of some responses to hepatotoxic insults. These common features include some or all of: persistent or intermittent hyperglycaemia, peripheral insulin resistance, hyperinsulinaemia, non-alcoholic fatty liver disease (NAFLD), central adiposity and ER stress in multiple tissues (Diamanti-Kandarakis and Dunaif 2012, Essah and Nestler 2006, Samuel and Shulman 2016, Tsatsoulis et al. 2013, Wainwright and Byrne 2016).

There seems little doubt that a major effect of supplemental Ins in most or all of these conditions is somehow to alleviate pathological insulin resistance (reviewed by Croze and Soulage 2013, Michell 2018). But we still do not know how Ins supplements bring about this effect – and this is also true of the insulin resensitization that is brought about by routine treatment of diabetes and metabolic syndrome with metformin (Rena, Hardie, and Pearson 2017).

Tokarz, MacDonald, and Klip (2018) have beautifully summarized the entire multi-organ choreography of insulin formation, action and destruction. Now we need to know on which parts of this endocrine ballet extra dietary Ins exerts its actions. However, most of the recent discussions of how eating extra Ins offers benefits in metabolic/endocrine diseases have diverged dramatically from modern mainstream views of insulin action, and of the ways in which this can become mis-regulated and/or faulty in disease.

On the one hand, it is now widely agreed that, downstream of the activated insulin receptor and its tyrosine-phosphorylated target proteins IRS1 and IRS2, two major and parallel signalling pathways lead to most or all cell responses, via: a) activation of PtdIns(3,4,5)P_3 synthesis by Type I phosphoinositide 3-kinase (PI3K-I); and b) Grb2-initiated activation of the MAP kinase pathway (Boucher, Kleinridders, and Kahn 2014, Choi and Kim 2010, Czech 2017, Lizcano and Alessi 2002).

By contrast, the commonly offered explanation for the therapeutic effects of eating inositol supplements (often *myo*-inositol alone, sometimes a *myo*-/D-*chiro*-inositol mixture and occasionally D-*chiro*-inositol alone) on insulin responsiveness is that the supplements support insulin signalling through two putative tissue-specific 'inositol phosphate glycan' (IPG) second messengers of insulin action, one of which contains *myo*-inositol and the other D-*chiro*-inositol (for recent discussions, see Croze and Soulage 2013, Larner, Brautigan, and Thorner 2010, Michell 2018). But the molecular details – and even the existence – of this third purported insulin signalling pathway remain unresolved almost 40 years after its original proposal. Moreover, the metabolism and possible functions of D-*chiro*-inositol (and derivatives thereof) remain so obscure that I shall not discuss them further, for reasons explained elsewhere (Michell 2018).

And then there is the mystery, highlighted by the strikingly different abundances of the various phosphoinositides (see Figure 1), of whether the cells in the organs of a mammal that has eaten quite a lot of Ins could ever channel the effects of this extra Ins intake selectively into the support of quantitatively very minor Ins-dependent metabolic pathway(s)? The central Ins-containing signalling molecules of the well-established PI 3-kinase/PtdIns(3,4,5)P_3/Akt insulin signalling pathway and of the still uncertain IPG second messenger-based signalling pathway are Ins lipids (or metabolites thereof) of very low abundance. These minor Ins derivatives will rarely, if ever, accumulate in cells to more than a small fraction of one percent of a cell's total phosphoinositide complement (Michell 2018). Despite this, none of the discussions of these ideas have ever tried to explain how the beneficial effects of a person eating 1-4 g of extra Ins each day – enough to more than double the usual dietary intake – might bring about highly *selective* effects on the levels and/or the functions of these rare Ins-containing constituents of eukaryote cells.

Possible Inter-Relationships between Intracellular Fat Accumulation, ER Stress and (Mal) Function, and Limitations on PtdIns Supply

The problem now is to assemble – from the miscellany of observations that has been briefly summarised above, in Table 1 and by Croze and Soulage (2013), Dinicola et al. (2017) and Michell (2018) – a clear picture of how dietary Ins supplements might: a) ameliorate fatty livers that are provoked in diverse ways; and b) counteract a variety of other endocrine and metabolic abnormalities in people and experimental animals. It must surely be sensible to search for a unitary hypothesis that might explain how a substantial extra systemic Ins supply ensures the unrestricted availability of some predominant and essential Ins-containing cell constituent, a plentiful supply of which is necessary for some central (but still unidentified) cell function(s)?

But which Ins-containing constituent and which functions(s)? The obvious candidate molecule is PtdIns, which is by far the cell's most abundant phosphoinositide (Figure 1). Much of this PtdIns is in the ER, but what does is it doing there and what might go wrong if a cell meets a challenge and finds itself without enough MI Ins and/or PtdIns to cope with the challenge? I recently suggested that expansion of the membrane area of the ER, which is needed both when the ER has to intensify its normal functions and as a part of its responses to other stresses, is a central cellular process that could readily be prejudiced by a less than dependable PtdIns supply, would be buttressed by eating Ins supplements, and might be the key cellular event in these responses (Michell 2018).

This idea tries to move us towards a unified explanation that might reconcile historical observations on experimental Ins deficiency with more recent work on the benefits of Ins supplements to patients, but its predictions are yet to be experimentally tested. Finally, therefore, I will briefly comment on how published studies of the liver, and especially of Ins-reversible accumulations of fat therein, have provided much of the evidence that led to this tentative proposal. This emphasis on events in the liver probably arose because fatty liver is an obvious phenotype and because the complex and constantly changing functions of this pivotal metabolic organ have been studied with unparalleled intensity. The functional impacts of limiting Ins supply to other organs may not be as immediately obvious, and they have been investigated much less. However, we should remember that they might be just as important and deserving of study (see, for example, Antony et al. 2017, Cnop, Foufelle, and Velloso 2012, Liu et al. 2014, Michell, 2018, Zammit 2013).

There are many situations, some of which were mentioned earlier and are listed in Table 1, in which fat droplets that consist mainly of triacylglycerol (TAG) accumulate within the ER membrane system of hepatocytes, and often also in other tissues. Many or all of these hepatic steatoses, maybe including the 'historical' fatty livers that were induced wholly or in part by Ins deficiency (Holub 1986, Michell 2018, Wells 1989) might nowadays travel under the more recently coined names of non-alcoholic fatty liver disease (NAFLD) (Henkel and Green 2013, Pagliassotti

2012) or toxicant-associated fatty liver disease (TAFLD) (Joshi-Barve et al. 2015, Wahlang et al. 2013). And these steatoses, which particularly involve the accumulation of lipid droplets in the ER, are inter-related in complex ways with various aspects of ER stress (see Basseri and Austin 2012, Dongiovanni et al. 2018, Fu, Watkins, and Hotamisligil 2012, Pagliassotti 2012, Pagliassotti et al. 2016).

The underlying mechanisms giving rise to such conditions are complex, and different balances of contributing factors are at play in different situations.

First, the fatty acids that are incorporated into fat droplets in hepatocytes, which mainly consist of triacylglycerols (TAGs), can have several origins and fates. Some fatty acids are liberated from dietary fat-derived chylomicra arriving in the chyle; some arrive in the bloodstream, having been released from 'overloaded' adipocytes; and some are locally made *de novo* from excess dietary carbohydrate by fatty acid synthase (FAS) (Zammit 2013).

Secondly, ER-associated fat droplets may serve as transient energy stores that accumulate and dissipate diurnally, tracking changes in an animal's nutritional status, or they may persist and enlarge over long periods, leading first to NAFLD and then potentially to its pathological sequelae (e.g., Cretenet, Le Clech, and Gachon 2010).

Thirdly, TAG that is initially laid down in these fat droplets may be re-mobilised, moved towards the Golgi apparatus and then reincorporated and packaged with cholesterol esters into the cores of apolipoprotein-stabilised very low density lipoprotein (VLDL) particles that are destined for exocytotic secretion.

Ins supplementation can ameliorate at least some of these apparently diverse 'fatty livers', apparently irrespective of whether they are caused by a deliberately induced Ins deficiency or by some other metabolic insult to the liver. However, the decline in research interest in overt Ins deficiency since the 1980s has meant that there has not been any systematic attempt to determine in how many of the diverse situations in which people or other animals exhibit conditions on the fatty liver/NAFLD/TAFLD spectrum they would gain benefit from consuming extra Ins – which is the reason for the 'at least some' vagueness of the statement at the start of this paragraph.

The exact aetiologies of these inter-related conditions are multifactorial (Joshi-Barve et al. 2015) but they seem to include – to varying degrees depending on the condition – a shared family of important contributing features: enhanced intra-hepatic generation of reactive oxygen species, with consequent oxidative stress; enhanced fatty acid mobilization from adipose tissue to the liver; increased acetyl-CoA carboxylase (ACC) and fatty acid synthase (FAS) activities, which feed newly synthesised palmitic acid into intra-hepatic triacylglycerol (TAG) droplet accumulation; slowing of the intracellular assembly, trafficking and secretion of VLDL particles by hepatocytes; various elements of the multifaceted ER stress responses; and tissue inflammation (see Dongiovanni et al. 2018, Fu, Watkins, and Hotamisligil 2012).

When we now look back to the 'classical' Ins deficiency studies of the 1970s and 1980s, we are reminded that they yielded an apparently sharp disagreement about what mechanism(s) led to the observed steatosis: was fat accumulation in the Ins-deficient liver caused by a delay in the secretion of assembled VLDL secretion from hepatocytes (Wells 1989) or did hepatocytes over-produce lipid droplets because of an 'excessive' hepatic influx of fatty acids that had been mobilised from adipose fat stores (Hayashi et al. 1978, Hayashi, Maeda, and Tomita 1974, Wells 1989)? We now know that both processes contribute to the causation of NAFLD, and it seems likely that this apparent dichotomy was false and that both processes contributed to the genesis of 'classical' Ins-deficient fatty livers – which would probably now have a new name: 'Ins deficiency-induced NAFLD'.

It seems clear that research to date has failed to explain either: a) the mechanisms that underlie the development and Ins-dependent resolution of Ins deficiency-induced NAFLD (because research on this problem was largely abandoned decades ago); or b) how Ins supplements ameliorate the manifestations of several metabolic/endocrine diseases (probably because interpretation of these clinical studies has tended to focus too obsessively on a less than proven model of insulin signalling). I recently suggested that the key to explaining both of these may lie in gaining an understanding of the particular role(s) that PtdIns plays in the function of the ER, and most notably its essential contribution to the increased ER membrane biosynthesis that is a central element of a cell's response to ER stress (Michell 2018). This idea remains to be tested.

Conflict of Interest

None

References

Abels, Jules C., Claudia W. Kupel, George T. Pack, and C. P. Rhoads. 1943. "Metabolic Studies in Patients with Cancer of Gastro-intestinal Tract. XV. Lipotropic Properties of Inositol." *Proceedings of the Society for Experimental Biology and Medicine* 54 (1):157-158.

Alb, James G., Scott E. Phillips, Lindsey R. Wilfley, Benjamin D. Philpot, and Vytas A. Bankaitis. 2007. "The pathologies associated with functional titration of phosphatidylinositol transfer protein α activity in mice." *Journal of Lipid Research* 48 (8):1857-1872.

Antony, Poovathumkal James, Gopalsamy Rajiv Gandhi, Antony Stalin, Kedike Balakrishna, Erenius Toppo, Kuppusamy Sivasankaran, Savarimuthu Ignacimuthu, and Naif Abdullah Al-Dhabi. 2017. "Myo-inositol ameliorates high-fat diet and streptozotocin-induced diabetes in rats through promoting insulin receptor signaling." *Biomedicine & Pharmacotherapy* 88:1098-1113.

Balla, Tamas. 2013. "Phosphoinositides: tiny lipids with giant impact on cell regulation." *Physiological Reviews* 93 (3):1019-1137.

Basseri, Sana, and Richard C. Austin. 2012. "Endoplasmic reticulum stress and lipid metabolism: mechanisms and therapeutic potential." *Biochemistry Research International:* (http://dx.doi.org/10.1155/2012/841362).

Beemster, Patricia, Pascal Groenen, and Régine Steegers-Theunissen. 2002. "Involvement of inositol in reproduction." *Nutrition reviews* 60 (3):80-87.

Bochud, Arlette, and Andreas Conzelmann. 2015. "The active site of yeast phosphatidylinositol synthase Pis1 is facing the cytosol." *Biochimica et Biophysica Acta (BBA)-Molecular and Cell Biology of Lipids* 1851 (5):629-640.

Boucher, Jérémie, André Kleinridders, and C. Ronald Kahn. 2014. "Insulin receptor signaling in normal and insulin-resistant states." *Cold Spring Harbor Perspectives in Biology* 6 (1):a009191.

Choi, Kangduk, and Young-Bum Kim. 2010. "Molecular mechanism of insulin resistance in obesity and type 2 diabetes." *The Korean journal of internal medicine* 25 (2):119-129.

Choy, Christopher H., Bong-Kwan Han, and Roberto J. Botelho. 2017. "Phosphoinositide diversity, distribution, and effector function: Stepping out of the box." *Bioessays* 39 (12): (https://doi.org/10.1002/bies.201700121)

Clark, Jonathan, Robert R. Kay, Anna Kielkowska, Izabella Niewczas, Louise Fets, David Oxley, Len R. Stephens, and Phillip T. Hawkins. 2014. "*Dictyostelium* uses ether-linked inositol phospholipids for intracellular signalling." *The EMBO Journal* 33 (19):2188-2200.

Clements Jr, Rex S., and Betty Darnell. 1980. "Myo-inositol content of common foods: development of a high-myo-inositol diet." *The American Journal of Clinical Nutrition* 33 (9):1954-1967.

Cnop, Miriam, Fabienne Foufelle, and Licio A. Velloso. 2012. "Endoplasmic reticulum stress, obesity and diabetes." *Trends in Molecular Medicine* 18 (1):59-68.

Cockcroft, Shamshad, and Padinjat Raghu. 2018. "Phospholipid transport protein function at organelle contact sites." *Current Opinion in Cell Biology* 53:52-60.

Cretenet, Gaspard, Mikaël Le Clech, and Frédéric Gachon. 2010. "Circadian clock-coordinated 12 hr period rhythmic activation of the IRE1α pathway controls lipid metabolism in mouse liver." *Cell Metabolism* 11 (1):47-57.

Croze, Marine L., and Christophe O. Soulage. 2013. "Potential role and therapeutic interests of myo-inositol in metabolic diseases." *Biochimie* 95 (10):1811-1827.

Czech, Michael P. 2017. "Insulin action and resistance in obesity and type 2 diabetes." *Nature Medicine* 23 (7):804-814.

Daughaday, William H., J. Larner, and Ellabeth Houghton. 1954. "The renal excretion of inositol by normal and diabetic rats." *The Journal of Clinical Investigation* 33 (8):1075-1080.

Di Paolo, Gilbert, and Pietro De Camilli. 2006. "Phosphoinositides in cell regulation and membrane dynamics." *Nature* 443 (7112):651-657.

Diamanti-Kandarakis, Evanthia, and Andrea Dunaif. 2012. "Insulin resistance and the polycystic ovary syndrome revisited: an update on mechanisms and implications." *Endocrine Reviews* 33 (6):981-1030.

Dinicola, Simona, Mirko Minini, Vittorio Unfer, Roberto Verna, Alessandra Cucina, and Mariano Bizzarri. 2017. "Nutritional and Acquired Deficiencies in Inositol Bioavailability. Correlations with Metabolic Disorders." *International Journal of Molecular Sciences* 18 (10):2187. (https://doi.org/10.3390/ijms18102187)

Dongiovanni, P., S. Stender, A. Pietrelli, R. M. Mancina, A. Cespiati, S. Petta, S. Pelusi, P. Pingitore, S. Badiali, and M. Maggioni. 2018. "Causal relationship of hepatic fat with liver damage and insulin resistance in nonalcoholic fatty liver." *Journal of Internal Medicine* 283 (4):356-370.

Dove, Stephen K., Kangzhen Dong, Takafumi Kobayashi, Fay K. Williams, and Robert H. Michell. 2009. "Phosphatidylinositol 3, 5-bisphosphate and Fab1p/PIKfyve underPPIn endo-lysosome function." *Biochemical Journal* 419 (1):1-13.

Duong, Q. H., K. G. Lapsley, and R. B. Pegg. 2018. "Inositol phosphates: health implications, methods of analysis and occurrence in plant foods." *J. Food Bioactives* 1:41-55.

English, Amber R., and Gia K. Voeltz. 2013. "Rab10 GTPase regulates ER dynamics and morphology." *Nature Cell Biology* 15 (2):169-178.

Essah, P. A., and J. E. Nestler. 2006. "The metabolic syndrome in polycystic ovary syndrome." *Journal of Endocrinological Investigation* 29 (3):270-280.

Fruman, David A., Honyin Chiu, Benjamin D. Hopkins, Shubha Bagrodia, Lewis C. Cantley, and Robert T. Abraham. 2017. "The PI3K pathway in human disease." *Cell* 170 (4):605-635. https://www.sciencedirect.com/science/article/pii/S0092867417308656

Fu, Suneng, Steven M. Watkins, and Gökhan S. Hotamisligil. 2012. "The role of endoplasmic reticulum in hepatic lipid homeostasis and stress signaling." *Cell Metabolism* 15 (5):623-634.

Greene, Nicholas D. E., and Andrew J. Copp. 1997. "Inositol prevents folate-resistant neural tube defects in the mouse." *Nature Medicine* 3 (1):60-66.

Greene, Nicholas D. E., Kit-Yi Leung, and Andrew J. Copp. 2017. "Inositol, neural tube closure and the prevention of neural tube defects." *Birth Defects Research* 109 (2):68-80.

Hallman, Mikko. 2015. "Inositol during perinatal transition." *Neo Reviews* 16 (2):e84-e93.

Hammond, Gerald R. V., and Tamas Balla. 2015. "Polyphosphoinositide binding domains: Key to inositol lipid biology." *Biochimica et Biophysica Acta (BBA)-Molecular and Cell Biology of Lipids* 1851 (6):746-758.

Hawthorne, J. N. 1960. "The inositol phospholipids." *Journal of Lipid Research* 1 (4):255-280.

Hayashi, E., T. Maeda, R. Hasegawa, and T. Tomita. 1978. "The effect of myo-inositol deficiency on lipid metabolism in rats: III. The mechanism of an enhancement in lipolysis due to myo-inositol deficiency in rats." *Biochimica et Biophysica Acta (BBA)-Lipids and Lipid Metabolism* 531 (2):197-205.

Hayashi, E., T. Maeda, and T. Tomita. 1974. "The effect of myo-inositol deficiency on lipid metabolism in rats: I. The alteration of lipid metabolism in myo-inositol deficient rats." *Biochimica et Biophysica Acta (BBA)-Lipids and Lipid Metabolism* 360 (2):134-145.

Henkel, Anne, and Richard M. Green. 2013. "The unfolded protein response in fatty liver disease." *Seminars in Liver Disease* 33(4): 321-329.

Ho, Cheuk Y., Tamadher A. Alghamdi, and Roberto J. Botelho. 2012. "Phosphatidylinositol-3,5-Bisphosphate: No Longer the Poor PIP2." *Traffic* 13 (1):1-8.

Holthuis, Joost C. M., and Anant K. Menon. 2014. "Lipid landscapes and pipelines in membrane homeostasis." *Nature* 510 (7503):48-57.

Holub, Bruce J. 1986. "Metabolism and function of myo-inositol and inositol phospholipids." *Annual Review of Nutrition* 6 (1):563-597.

Hong, Jun Hwa, Hye Won Jang, Yea Eun Kang, Ju Hee Lee, Koon Soon Kim, Hyun Jin Kim, Kyu Ri Park, and Bon Jeong Ku. 2012. "Urinary *chiro*-and *myo*-inositol levels as a biological marker for type 2 diabetes mellitus." *Disease Markers* 33 (4):193-199.

Idevall-Hagren, Olof, and Pietro De Camilli. 2015. "Detection and manipulation of phosphoinositides." *Biochimica et Biophysica Acta (BBA)-Molecular and Cell Biology of Lipids* 1851 (6):736-745.

Irvine, Robin F. 2016. "A short history of inositol lipids." *Journal of Lipid Research* 57 (11):1987-1994.

Irvine, Robin F., Simon J. Bulley, Miranda S. Wilson, and Adolfo Saiardi. 2015. "There is no 'Conundrum' of $InsP_6$." *Open Biology* 5 (11):150181.

Joshi-Barve, Swati, Irina Kirpich, Matthew C. Cave, Luis S. Marsano, and Craig J. McClain. 2015. "Alcoholic, nonalcoholic, and toxicant-associated steatohepatitis: mechanistic similarities and differences." *Cellular and Molecular Gastroenterology and Hepatology* 1 (4):356-367.

Joshi, Amit S., Hong Zhang, and William A. Prinz. 2017. "Organelle biogenesis in the endoplasmic reticulum." *Nature Cell Biology* 19 (8):876-882.

Kawa, Julianne M., Roman Przybylski, and Carla G. Taylor. 2003. "Urinary *chiro*-inositol and *myo*-inositol excretion is elevated in the diabetic db/db mouse and streptozotocin diabetic rat." *Experimental Biology and Medicine* 228 (8):907-914.

Kim, Yeun Ju, Maria-Luisa Guzman Hernandez, and Tamas Balla. 2013. "Inositol lipid regulation of lipid transfer in specialized membrane domains." *Trends in Cell Biology* 23 (6):270-278.

Kuksis, A., and S. Mookerjea. 1978. "Inositol." *Nutrition Reviews* 36 (8):233-238.

Larner, Joseph, David L. Brautigan, and Michael O. Thorner. 2010. "D-chiro-inositol glycans in insulin signaling and insulin resistance." *Molecular Medicine* 16 (11-12):543-552.

Lemmon, Mark A. 2008. "Membrane recognition by phospholipid-binding domains." *Nature Reviews Molecular Cell Biology* 9 (2):99.

Liu, Yuan, Wei Wang, Guanghou Shui, and Xun Huang. 2014. "CDP-diacylglycerol synthetase coordinates cell growth and fat storage through phosphatidylinositol metabolism and the insulin pathway." *PLoS Genetics* 10 (3):e1004172.

Lizcano, Jose M., and Dario R. Alessi. 2002. "The insulin signalling pathway." *Current Biology* 12 (7):R236-R238.

Michell, Robert H. 2008. "Inositol derivatives: evolution and functions." *Nature Reviews Molecular Cell Biology* 9 (2):151-161.

Michell, Robert H. 2018. "Do inositol supplements enhance phosphatidylinositol supply and thus support endoplasmic reticulum function?" *British Journal of Nutrition* 120 (3):1-16.

Morii, Hiroyuki, Midori Ogawa, Kazumasa Fukuda, and Hatsumi Taniguchi. 2014. "Ubiquitous distribution of phosphatidylinositol phosphate synthase and archaetidylinositol phosphate synthase in Bacteria and Archaea, which contain inositol phospholipid." *Biochemical and Biophysical Research Communications* 443 (1):86-90.

Murphy, Aisling, Amir Shamshirsaz, Daniela Markovic, Richard Ostlund, and Brian Koos. 2016. "Urinary excretion of *myo*-inositol and d-*chiro*-inositol in early pregnancy is enhanced in gravidas with gestational diabetes mellitus." *Reproductive Sciences* 23 (3):365-371.

Nayak, Baibaswata, Vinay K. Kondeti, Ping Xie, Sun Lin, Navin Vishwakarma, Kirtee Raparia, and Yashpal S. Kanwar. 2011. "Transcriptional and post-translational modulation of *myo*-inositol oxygenase by high glucose and related pathobiological stresses." *Journal of Biological Chemistry* 286 (31):27594-275611.

Nishigaki, Ikuo, Syed H. Hasan, Akira Kotaki, Kunio Yagi, Sumihiko Okuyama, Shozo Ito, Kozo Yamada, and Kazuo Yamashita. 1971. "Studies on Myoinositol." *The Journal of Vitaminology* 17 (2):112-116.

Nishimura, Taki, Norito Tamura, Nozomu Kono, Yuta Shimanaka, Hiroyuki Arai, Hayashi Yamamoto, and Noboru Mizushima. 2017. "Autophagosome formation is initiated at phosphatidylinositol synthase-enriched ER subdomains." *The EMBO Journal* 36 (12):1719-1735.

Pagliassotti, Michael J. 2012. "Endoplasmic reticulum stress in nonalcoholic fatty liver disease." *Annual Review of Nutrition* 32:17-33.

Pagliassotti, Michael J., Paul Y. Kim, Andrea L. Estrada, Claire M. Stewart, and Christopher L. Gentile. 2016. "Endoplasmic reticulum stress in obesity and obesity-related disorders: An expanded view." *Metabolism* 65 (9):1238-1246.

Pak, Yunbae, Charles R. Paule, Yong-Dae Bao, Laura C. Huang, and Joseph Larner. 1993. "Insulin stimulates the biosynthesis of *chiro*-inositol-containing phospholipids in a rat fibroblast line expressing the human insulin receptor." *Proceedings of the National Academy of Sciences* 90 (16):7759-7763.

Rena, Graham, D. Grahame Hardie, and Ewan R. Pearson. 2017. "The mechanisms of action of metformin." *Diabetologia* 60 (9):1577-1585.

Ryals, Phillip E., and Michael C. Kersting. 1999. "Sodium-dependent uptake of [^{3}H]*scyllo*-inositol by *Tetrahymena*: incorporation into phosphatidylinositol, phosphatidylinositol-linked glycans, and polyphosphoinositols." *Archives of Biochemistry and Biophysics* 366 (2):261-266.

Samuel, Varman T., and Gerald I. Shulman. 2016. "The pathogenesis of insulin resistance: integrating signaling pathways and substrate flux." *The Journal of Clinical Investigation* 126 (1):12-22.

Schlemmer, Ulrich, Wenche Frølich, Rafel M. Prieto, and Felix Grases. 2009. "Phytate in foods and significance for humans: food sources, intake, processing, bioavailability, protective role and analysis." *Molecular Nutrition & Food Research* 53 (S2):S330-S375.

Stefan, Christopher J., William S. Trimble, Sergio Grinstein, Guillaume Drin, Karin Reinisch, Pietro De Camilli, Sarah Cohen, Alex M. Valm, Jennifer Lippincott-Schwartz, and Tim P. Levine. 2017. "Membrane dynamics and organelle biogenesis—lipid pipelines and vesicular carriers." *BMC Biology* 15 (1):102. doi.org/10.1186/s12915-017-0432-0

Thakur, Prakash C., Jon M. Davison, Carsten Stuckenholz, Lili Lu, and Nathan Bahary. 2014. "Dysregulated phosphatidylinositol signaling promotes endoplasmic-reticulum-stress-mediated intestinal mucosal injury and inflammation in zebrafish." *Disease Models & Mechanisms* 7 (1):93-106.

Thakur, Prakash C., Carsten Stuckenholz, Marcus R. Rivera, Jon M. Davison, Jeffrey K. Yao, Adam Amsterdam, Kirsten C. Sadler, and Nathan Bahary. 2011. "Lack of *de novo* phosphatidylinositol synthesis leads to endoplasmic reticulum stress and hepatic steatosis in cdipt-deficient zebrafish." *Hepatology* 54 (2):452-462.

Tokarz, Victoria L., Patrick E. MacDonald, and Amira Klip. 2018. "The cell biology of systemic insulin function." *Journal of Cell Biology* 217 (7):2273-2289.

Tominaga, Tatsuya, Rajesh K. Dutta, Darukeshwara Joladarashi, Toshio Doi, Janardan K. Reddy, and Yashpal S. Kanwar. 2015. "Transcriptional and Translational Modulation of *myo*-Inositol Oxygenase (Miox) by Fatty Acids: Implications in renal tubular injury induced in obesity and diabetes." *Journal of Biological Chemistry.* 291 (3): 1348-1367.

Tsatsoulis, Agathocles, Michalis D. Mantzaris, Sofia Bellou, and Maria Andrikoula. 2013. "Insulin resistance: an adaptive mechanism becomes maladaptive in the current environment—an evolutionary perspective." *Metabolism* 62 (5):622-633.

Vucenik, Ivana, and AbulKalam M. Shamsuddin. 2006. "Protection against cancer by dietary IP6 and inositol." *Nutrition and Cancer* 55 (2):109-125.

Wahlang, Banrida, Juliane I. Beier, Heather B. Clair, Heather J. Bellis-Jones, K. Cameron Falkner, Craig J. McClain, and Matt C. Cave. 2013. "Toxicant-associated steatohepatitis." *Toxicologic Pathology* 41 (2):343-360.

Wainwright, Patrick, and Christopher D. Byrne. 2016. "Bidirectional relationships and disconnects between NAFLD and features of the metabolic syndrome." *International Journal of Molecular Sciences 17*(3), 367; doi:10.3390/ijms17030367

Wallroth, Alexander, and Volker Haucke. 2017. "Phosphoinositide conversion in endocytosis and the endolysosomal system." *Journal of Biological Chemistry* 293, 1526-1535.

Wells, William W. 1989. "Inositol deficiency states as a guide to inositol function." In *Inositol Lipids in Cell Signalling* (Robert H. Michell, Alan H. Drummond, and C. Peter Downes, eds.) pp. 209-238, Academic Press, London.

Williams, Tom A., and T. Martin Embley. 2015. Changing ideas about eukaryotic origins. *Philosophical Transactions of the Royal Society, Series B* 370(1678):20140318. doi: 10.1098/rstb.2014.0318.

Wong, Louise H., Alenka Čopič, and Tim P. Levine. 2017. "Advances on the transfer of lipids by lipid transfer proteins." *Trends in Biochemical Sciences* 42 (7):516-530.

Woolley, D. W. 1941. "A study of the biological specificity of inositol." *Journal of Biological Chemistry* 140:461-466.

Yang, Bingmei, Andrea Hodgkinson, Beverley A. Millward, and Andrew G. Demaine. 2010. "Polymorphisms of myo-inositol oxygenase gene are associated with Type 1 diabetes mellitus." *Journal of Diabetes and Its Complications* 24 (6):404-408.

Zammit, Victor A. 2013. "Hepatic triacylglycerol synthesis and secretion: DGAT2 as the link between glycaemia and triglyceridaemia." *Biochemical Journal* 451 (1):1-12.

Zurzolo, Chiara, and Kai Simons. 2016. "Glycosylphosphatidylinositol-anchored proteins: Membrane organization and transport." *Biochimica et Biophysica Acta (BBA)-Biomembranes* 1858 (4):632-639.

In: Inositols
Editor: Vittorio Unfer
ISBN: 978-1-53614-912-8

Chapter 3

INOSITOLS IN POLYCYSTIC OVARY SYNDROME

Morgan Vargo[1], MD, Stéphanie B. Mayer[1,2,*], MD and John E. Nestler[1], MD

[1]Virginia Commonwealth University, Division of Endocrinology, Diabetes and Metabolism. Richmond, VA, US

[2]Hunter Holmes McGuire VA Medical Center, Division of Endocrinology and Metabolism, Richmond, VA, US

ABSTRACT

Polycystic ovary syndrome (PCOS), affecting 5-10% of women of reproductive age (Knochenhauer, E. S. 1998), is a prevalent disorder defined by chronic anovulation and hyperandrogenism leading to infertility. PCOS affects both lean and obese women. Insulin resistance is a prominent feature in most women with PCOS. Thus far, metformin has been recommended for treatment of PCOS to increase ovulation, reduce serum androgen levels, and improve hirsutism (Nestler, J. E., 2008). More recently, inositols have been identified as insulin sensitizers and are

* Corresponding Author's Email: stephanie.mayer@vcuhealth.org.

considered for the treatment of PCOS, particularly for restoration of ovulation and fertility.

Keywords: inositol, myo-inositol, d-chiro-inositol, polycystic ovary syndrome, PCOS

Methods

A review of the literature was performed in PubMed and Embase using keywords and controlled vocabulary for the concepts polycystic ovarian syndrome and inositol. The following representative search was used in PubMed and then adapted to Embase: ("Polycystic Ovary Syndrome"[Mesh] OR "polycystic ovary" OR "polycystic ovarian" OR PCOS[tiab]) AND ("Inositol"[Mesh] OR "Inositol"[nm] OR inositol OR inositols OR myo-inositol OR "myo inositol" OR "D chiro inositol" OR "D chiroinositol"). An additional search of the grey literature was performed through Web of Science. We also had direct communication with one of the lead authors of a scientific article where noted in the citation.

Introduction

Definition of PCOS

Polycystic Ovary Syndrome (PCOS) remains a clinical diagnosis. Diagnosis of PCOS requires a thorough clinical and biochemical evaluation of the patient to document the degree of hyperandrogenism present and to exclude alternative causes of oligo- amenorrhea or androgen excess, including pregnancy, hyperprolactinemia, hyper- or hypothyroidism, non-classical congenital adrenal hyperplasia, androgen-secreting ovarian or adrenal tumors, premature ovarian insufficiency, hypogonadotrophic hypogonadism, and hypercortisolemia. Several different medical conferences and societies (1990 NIH expert conference, 2003 Rotterdam statement, and the Androgen Excess Society) have published guidelines on the definition of PCOS since the original publication by Stein and Leventhal in 1935, which described women with chronic anovulation associated with androgen excess (Azziz et al. 2009, Rotterdam 2004, Zawadzki 1992, Stein and Leventhal 1935).

The androgen excess of PCOS may be visible as the combination phenotype of hirsutism, seborrhea, acne, alopecia and occasionally virilization of the external genitalia. Guidelines have evolved as it has become clear that there is a spectrum of presentations of PCOS, namely both lean and obese women who have varying degrees of clinical or biochemical hyperandrogenism. As technologies and assays have advanced, the definition of PCOS has subsequently continued to evolve.

Currently the most frequently cited diagnostic criteria for PCOS are the 2003 Rotterdam guidelines which require the exclusion of secondary causes of androgen excess or oligo-ovulation and the presence of at least two out of the following three criteria: 1) chronic oligo- or anovulation 2) clinical or biochemical signs of hyperandrogenism, or 3) polycystic ovaries on ultra sonographic imaging, noting that the specific numerical and size cutoffs for defining polycystic ovaries continue to evolve as ultrasonography technology evolves as well. Typically, the most common causes of secondary oligomenorrhea or androgen excess that are excluded are thyroid disorders, adrenal hyperplasia and hyperprolactinemia.

Insulin and Metabolic Comorbidities

Insulin, and more specifically insulin resistance with its resultant hyperinsulinemia, is a prominent feature in a majority of women with PCOS, and appears to be integral to its underlying pathophysiology, preceding, and likely causative of, the resultant hyperandrogenic state, regardless of body mass index (BMI). Increasing insulin levels lead to increasing levels of circulating androgens, both by stimulating ovarian biosynthesis and secretion of testosterone, and by suppressing hepatic production of the major binding protein of testosterone in circulation, sex hormone binding globulin

(SHBG). Lower levels of SHBG in circulation result in higher levels of circulating free testosterone. The presence of insulin resistance is observed in women with PCOS independently of the presence or absence of obesity (Dunaif et al. 1989).

Women with PCOS are at increased risk of developing comorbidities associated with insulin resistance such as impaired glucose tolerance (IGT), diabetes mellitus, and metabolic syndrome, at an earlier age, than age matched cohorts who do not have PCOS. A prospective controlled trial (n = 144), demonstrated that among women with PCOS, at baseline 37% had IGT and 10% had type 2 diabetes. Over 2-3 years of follow-up, 16% converted each year from normal glucose tolerance to IGT and 2% converted each year from IGT to diabetes mellitus type 2 (DM2) (Legro et al. 1999).

Further, women with PCOS develop early signs of atherosclerotic disease at an earlier age (Birdsall, Farquhar, and White 1997, Orio et al. 2004). Notably, in a study of young (mean age 22 years old) lean (mean BMI 22 kg/m2) women with PCOS (n = 30) without cardiovascular disease (CVD), compared to age and BMI-matched control women without PCOS, the women with PCOS demonstrated impaired flow-mediated dilation, accompanied by an increased serum endothelin-1 level, and increased intima-media thickness of the carotid arteries. These young, lean women with PCOS were already showing anatomic and functional cardiac abnormalities (Orio et al. 2004).

In terms of cardiovascular outcomes, Mani et al. reported that in a 20-year retrospective study of 2,301 women with PCOS in England totaling >12,000 person-years, the prevalence of myocardial infarction in the age group 45–54 was 1.9%, age 55–64 was 6.0% and >65 years 27.3%. Prevalence of angina symptoms similarly up trended by age (age 45–54 was 2.6%, age 55–64 was 6.0% and >65 years was 27.3%). The prevalence of these age-specific cardiovascular events were significantly higher in the women with PCOS when compared to the local population or to the population of women in England as a whole (Mani et al. 2012). In accordance with these findings, the Nurses' Health Study, published in 2002, followed 82,439 women in the United States for 14 years, and found that in women with very irregular periods the risk ratio for coronary heart disease was 1.5 and there was a 2-fold increase in the risk for fatal myocardial infarction (Solomon et al. 2002). Since 50-80% of women who experience fewer than or equal to 8 menses annually have PCOS, chronic oligomenorrhea is a fair surrogate marker for PCOS.

Treatment of Insulin Resistance

Targeting amelioration of peripheral insulin resistance has been an area of active research in the treatment of PCOS for the past two decades. The main thrust of this research has been focused on the use of the insulin-sensitizing drug metformin, as well as dietary interventions that improve insulin resistance. Dietary interventions should accompany any pharmacologic treatment because weight loss of 5-10% can restore ovulation in approximately 50% of patients with PCOS. As an insulin-sensitizing agent, metformin has been shown to reduce progression to IGT and to DM2 (Sharma, Wickham, and Nestler 2007). Metformin is thought to improve infertility in women with PCOS indirectly by improving insulin sensitivity.

As an example, in a study by Diamanti-Kandarakis et al. in 1998, 16 obese women with PCOS were treated with metformin for 6 months; insulin sensitivity was assessed by the euglycemic-hyperinsulinemic clamp technique at baseline and end-of-study (Diamanti-Kandarakis et al. 1998). After 6 months of metformin therapy, the authors found that glucose utilization and insulin action had improved, and that this was accompanied by significant increases in the serum levels of SHBG and decreases in serum free testosterone and androstenedione levels. Among these women with PCOS, 44% resumed normal cycles and two cases of spontaneous pregnancy occurred during treatment with metformin.

By improving peripheral insulin sensitivity and reducing circulating insulin levels, it is theorized that intra-ovarian concentrations of androgens will decrease. Additionally, there is a reduction in GnRH-stimulated LH release, mediated perhaps by improvement in insulin sensitivity at the hypothalamus or pituitary, or through a reduction in circulating insulin levels (Nestler et al. 1999). Recent attention has focused on the role of elevated anti-Mullerian hormone (AMH) in PCOS. AMH levels are often elevated 2 to 3-fold higher in women with PCOS. Foroozanfard et al. assessed AMH levels in 30 women with PCOS and infertility after treatment for 8 weeks with 1,500 mg of metformin daily and found that AMH levels decreased significantly and were directly associated with BMI (Foroozanfard et al. 2017).

The 2017 American Society for Reproductive Medicine Practice Committee consensus states that metformin compared to placebo does increase ovulation rates in women with PCOS, but that the ovulation induction agents clomiphene citrate or letrozole are first line therapy when comparing efficacy of live birth rates in women with PCOS. They proceed to state that at the current writing there is insufficient data to state that metformin in combination with other agents increases live birth rates, and that this remains an area to be investigated (Penzias 2017).

Tissue Specific Insulin Sensitivity – Ovarian Paradox

There is a phenomenon of tissue-specific insulin resistance in women with PCOS that has been termed the "ovarian insulin paradox in PCOS." That is, a differential range of sensitivity and resistance to insulin is found at different tissues in women with PCOS. In women with PCOS, the ovaries remain sensitive to the effects of insulin even while peripheral insulin target tissues (such as muscle, fat and liver) manifest profound insulin resistance. Though seemingly paradoxical, at the level of the ovarian thecal cell, insulin continues to stimulate steroidogenesis and androgen secretion in women with PCOS, in spite of the fact that the peripheral tissues of these women are resistant to insulin (Willis and Franks 1995).

As will be outlined below, the fact that the ovary maintains normal insulin sensitivity in women with PCOS, even while classic insulin target tissues manifest profound insulin resistance, has important implications for the intracellular metabolism of inositols.

Inositols

Coming to the forefront recently has been the use of inositols, specifically D-chiroinositol (DCI) or Myo-inositol (MI), or a combination of the two inositols, for the treatment of insulin resistance and infertility in women diagnosed with PCOS. Inositols are sugar alcohols typically found in our diet. An additional source of DCI is derived from the intracellular conversion of MI to DCI by an epimerase enzyme. It is important to note that the activity of this epimerase enzyme is stimulated by insulin.

The inositols are converted intracellularly to inositolphosphoglycan (IPG) second messengers of insulin action. These IPGs are anchored on the outside of the cells, and through a G-protein mediated process are released when insulin binds to its receptor. The IPGs then act in paracrine and autocrine fashion to mediate some of the effects of insulin. The MI-containing IPG (MI-IPG) is primarily involved in cellular glucose uptake, whereas the DCI-containing IPG (DCI-IPG) is primarily involved in glycogen synthesis (Figure 1).

Low levels of DCI have been demonstrated in the urine of insulin-resistant subjects, such as individuals with IGT, diabetes and PCOS. Moreover, a decrease in the release of the DCI-IPG during an oral glucose tolerance test has been reported in muscle of subjects with diabetes (Asplin, Galasko, and Larner 1993, Kennington et al. 1990). Conversely, the administration of DCI to insulin-resistant monkeys was demonstrated to enhance glucose disposal, presumably reflecting enhanced insulin sensitivity (Larner 2002). Based on these findings and their insulin-mimetic actions, the inositols surfaced as promising candidate agents for the treatment of PCOS.

MI and DCI are the two stereoisomers that have been clinically studied. As noted earlier, intracellularly DCI is formed from MI by an epimerase enzyme, which is stimulated by insulin (Figure 2). MI and DCI have different roles: MI regulates cellular glucose uptake and FSH signaling, while DCI is involved in glycogen synthesis and appears to modulate insulin-stimulated thecal androgen synthesis (Nestler et al. 1991). Based on each molecule's respective function, it is not surprising that they are found in varying concentrations in different target tissues. DCI levels are high in glycogen storage tissues such as liver, muscle, and fat, and low in tissues with high glucose utilization such as the brain, heart, and ovary (Nestler et al. 1991). Additionally, there appear to be tissue specific ratios of MI : DCI. In the serum of normal healthy women, the MI : DCI ratio is 40 : 1. To date, the serum MI : DCI ratio in women with PCOS has not been reported. In the follicular fluid of the ovary, the MI : DCI ratio in healthy women is 100:1, while in women with PCOS who are hyperinsulinemic the MI : DCI ratio is reversed to 0.2 : 1, due to much lower MI content and higher DCI content (Unfer et al. 2014).

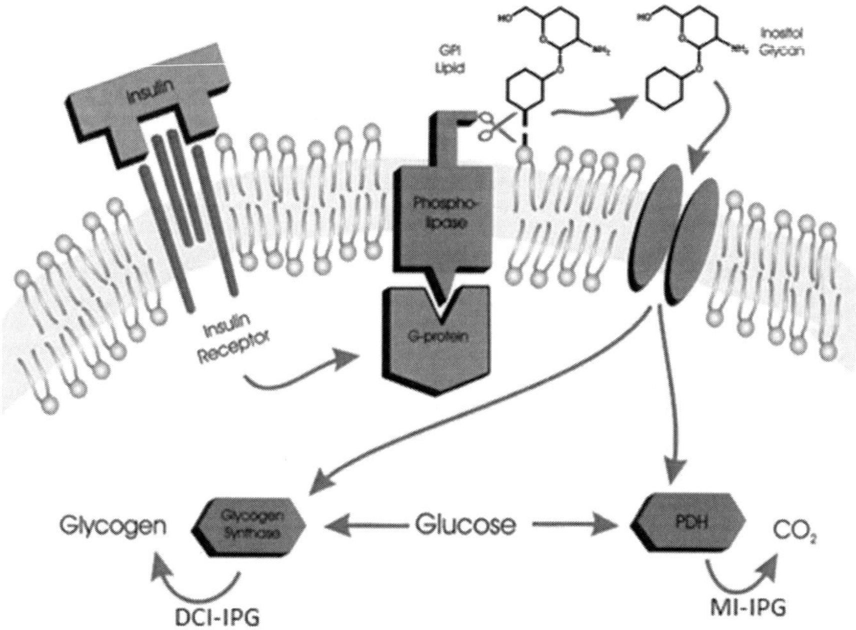

Figure 1. Inositolphosphoglycan (IPG) mediators of insulin action are located on the outside of cells and anchored in the cellular membrane. When insulin binds to its receptor, a phospholipase is activated through a G-protein process, and the activated phospholipase then cleaves the IPG from its anchor. The IPG can then either enter its own cell (autocrine action) or a neighboring cell (paracrine action) and mediate insulin actions. D-chiroinositol phosphoglycan (DCI-IPG) stimulates glycogen synthase and Myo-inositol phosphoglycan (MI-IPG) stimulates pyruvate dehydrogenase.

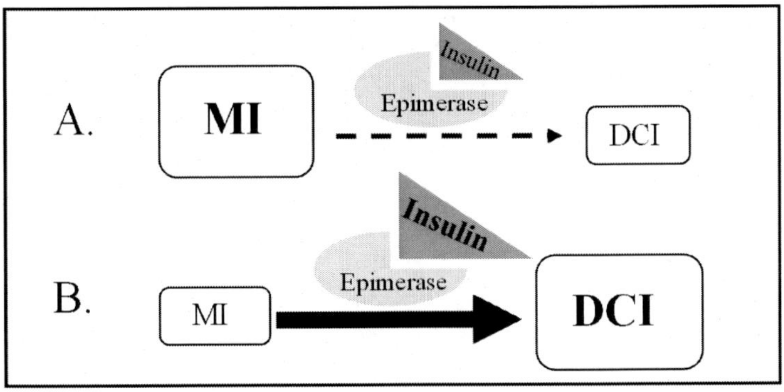

Figure 2. The epimerase enzyme responsible for conversion of myo-inositol (MI) to D-chiroinositol (DCI) is stimulated by insulin. In women with polycystic ovary syndrome (PCOS) and insulin resistance there is compensatory hyperinsulinemia to maintain normal glucose levels. A) In classic insulin target tissues there is less epimerase activity due to insulin resistance. B) The ovary maintains normal insulin sensitivity and therefore is hyperstimulated by the higher circulating insulin concentration.

An explanation for the altered ratio of MI : DCI in the ovaries of women with PCOS is the fact that, contrary to the peripheral insulin resistance inherent to PCOS, the ovaries in women with PCOS still maintain normal insulin sensitivity (Willis and Franks 1995). This has been termed the 'ovarian paradox' as described above. When the epimerase enzyme in the ovary is exposed to higher levels of insulin, as is the case in PCOS, the activity of the epimerase enzyme is subsequently increased (Heimark, McAllister, and Larner 2014). This results in enhanced epimerase conversion of MI to DCI in the ovaries resulting in a depletion of MI, and a rise in DCI levels in the ovary of women with PCOS (Figure 2).

As a result of the stimulated epimerase activity in the ovary, there is an altered ratio of MI : DCI in the follicular fluid of women with PCOS, reflecting depletion of MI (Unfer et al. 2014). As the dominant intracellular inositol in the normal ovary, MI plays an important role in follicle development and oocyte quality (Chiu et al. 2002). MI depletion at the ovary in women with PCOS likely contributes to the infertility associated with PCOS through impaired folliculogenesis, as reflected by decreased frequency of ovulation and reduced oocyte quality.

Treatment with Inositols in PCOS

Since alterations in inositol metabolism likely play a role in the pathophysiology of PCOS, both MI and DCI have been considered potential treatment options for PCOS. They have been investigated for a variety of outcomes including improvement in insulin sensitivity, reduction in serum testosterone, and for improved ovulatory rates and fertility. Supplementation with low dose DCI (1,200 mg daily) improved both ovulatory frequency and the metabolic abnormalities of PCOS, presumably by altering the degree of peripheral insulin resistance and decreasing circulating insulin levels. In two studies of 22 and 20 patients with PCOS, respectively, administration of low dose DCI improved ovulatory function, decreased serum and ovarian androgen levels, lowered cholesterol levels and improved blood pressure (Iuorno et al. 2002, Nestler et al. 1999). It was posited that the improvement in ovarian function from administration of DCI was likely due to the reduction in circulating insulin, thereby decreasing effects of insulin on the ovary. As mentioned earlier, the ovary maintains normal insulin sensitivity; therefore, a reduction in serum insulin results in reduced intra-ovarian epimerase activity, thus reducing conversion of MI to DCI in the ovary. This indirect effect should then restore the MI concentration and MI : DCI balance towards normal, positively affecting oocyte maturation and FSH signaling.

When higher doses of DCI (2,400 mg daily) were administered, it was actually found to be detrimental to ovulation and follicle development (Isabella and Raffone 2012). The explanation for this conflicting observation is unclear, although it may be due to DCI-IPG mediated stimulation of androgen secretion (Nestler et al. 1991).

Several studies using MI alone have been performed in women with PCOS. They focused on reproductive outcomes, including ovulation rates and oocyte quality. It was hypothesized that the deficiency of MI in the ovary of women with PCOS contributes to poor follicle health and blighted folliculogenesis. It was demonstrated that MI supplementation at doses of 2,000-4,000 mg daily improved spontaneous ovulation in women with PCOS, with a decrease in time to first ovulation (Gerli et al. 2007). In women with PCOS undergoing in vitro fertilization, administration of MI reduced the number of FSH injections necessary per cycle and improved both oocyte quality and implantation rate (Artini et al. 2017, Papaleo et al. 2009). MI supplementation also reduced serum insulin levels and improved insulin sensitivity (Genazzani et al. 2008). Additional studies are needed to draw conclusions about the effects of MI alone on metabolic parameters because these were often secondary outcomes and the findings were mixed. Collectively, however, the administration of MI to women with PCOS appears to improve peripheral insulin sensitivity and reduce serum testosterone levels (Costantino et al. 2009). In addition to these studies, a meta-analysis of nine articles assessing fasting insulin concentrations in women with PCOS after the use of MI or DCI showed a significant decrease in fasting insulin levels and insulin resistance in those treated with MI compared to controls. Additionally, there was a non-significant trend toward a reduction in testosterone levels for those treated with MI (Unfer et al. 2017).

With a combined goal of improving both infertility and the metabolic syndrome associated with PCOS, MI in combination with DCI has been investigated as a therapeutic combination. A trial was conducted in 50 women with PCOS, who were randomized to either MI alone (2,000 mg daily in powder form) or to combination MI+DCI (550 mg MI plus 13.8 mg DCI in gel capsule) in a ratio designed to mimic the normal physiologic serum ratio of MI : DCI of 40 : 1. Analysis at 3 months demonstrated significant reductions in fasting plasma glucose and insulin concentrations and glucose-stimulated insulin levels in the women treated with MI+DCI. After 6 months of treatment however, there was no significant difference in plasma glucose or insulin concentration between the groups, suggesting that the combination treatment of MI+DCI may result in metabolic improvements more rapidly than MI alone. The combination treatment of MI+DCI resulted in a greater decrease in serum testosterone and increase in SHBG levels at both the three month and 6-month time points than MI alone, although the differences did not attain statistical significance. All women in the study, who at baseline had a mean of 3 menstrual cycles per year, ovulated based on reaching serum progesterone levels greater than 10 ng/mL (measured weekly) regardless of group assignment and with no statistical difference in ovulation rates (Nordio and Proietti 2012) (additional data obtained from direct communication with lead author Professor Maurizio Nordio).

A second trial of 100 women with PCOS undergoing in vitro fertilization were randomly assigned to receive either MI+DCI (550 mg MI + 13.8 mg DCI twice daily) or low dose DCI alone (500 mg twice daily). Women who received MI+DCI required less recombinant FSH for ovarian stimulation and had lower estradiol levels before HCG administration. The MI+DCI group also yielded better oocyte quality with fewer degenerated oocytes, which led to improved fertilization rates (Colazingari et al. 2013). This study, as well as that of Nordio and colleagues above, demonstrated enhanced benefit for both metabolic and reproduction outcomes with the use of MI and DCI in combination (at a ratio of 40 : 1) versus either inositol alone.

In a longitudinal uncontrolled study of 20 obese Caucasian women with PCOS treated with 550 mg MI + 13.8 mg DCI twice daily for 6 months, several positive effects on markers of metabolic health were observed, including lower LDL-c levels, increased levels of HDL-c, improved insulin sensitivity and a decrease in fasting insulin and glucose levels (Minozzi, Nordio, and Pajalich 2013). Additionally, a randomized trial of 46 women with PCOS receiving either MI+DCI in the 40 : 1 ratio (550 mg MI plus 13.8 mg DCI and folic acid twice daily) or placebo (folic acid alone) reported a significant reduction in LH and free testosterone in the group treated with MI+DCI, as well as a significant increase in estradiol and SHBG levels as compared to folic acid supplementation alone. The combination treatment of MI+DCI also resulted in improvements in insulin resistance as reduced fasting glucose and HOMA index (Benelli et al. 2016).

Metformin versus Inositols

In a study of 120 women with PCOS randomly assigned to metformin 1,500 mg/day or MI 4,000 mg daily, plus folic acid, there was no significant difference between groups in the rate of ovulation or number of pregnancies (Raffone, Rizzo, and Benedetto 2010), hence suggesting equivalency. In this regard, an interesting observation is that some of the beneficial effects of metformin itself may relate to its ability to enhance insulin-mediated release of the DCI-IPG mediator (Baillargeon et al. 2004). In a second study of 60 women with PCOS, who were randomized to receive either metformin 1,500 mg/day or MI 4,000 mg plus folic acid after 12 weeks of treatment, MI, as compared to metformin, showed a significantly greater decrease in serum total testosterone and Ferriman-Gallwey scores, as well as a lower high sensitivity C-reactive protein and reduced gene expression of interleukin-1 (Jamilian, et al. 2017). In a third study of 26 obese women with PCOS treated with metformin 850 mg twice daily or MI 1,000mg twice daily for 6 months with a crossover design, only treatment with metformin significantly decreased body weight, improved menstrual cycle frequency, Ferriman-Gallwey scores, decreased LH, estradiol, and androstenedione levels. During treatment with either metformin or MI, there was significant reduction in the insulin response to oral glucose tolerance testing (Tagliaferri, V., et al. 2017). This study suggests that both metformin and MI impact insulin resistance; however, metformin has greater effect on weight reduction for obese women with PCOS. Lastly, a randomized control trial of women with PCOS (n=50) affected by insulin resistance and/or hyperinsulinemia were treated with either metformin 1,500 mg/day or MI 4,000 mg/day plus folic acid and compared to a control group of healthy women with normal menstrual cycles and no symptoms of hyperandrogenism. Women in both treatment groups showed a significant reduction in BMI and improvement in insulin resistance with no difference between the two groups. This study suggests that MI is as effective as metformin in improving the metabolic profile of women with PCOS (Fruzzetti, F., et al. 2016). Although, there is heterogeneity in the results, there is a role for the use of MI in the treatment of metabolic disease and infertility in women with PCOS, especially for those who are unable to tolerate metformin due to gastrointestinal side effects.

Conclusion

The inositols MI and DCI are important treatment considerations in PCOS, especially for the gynecologist when the patient's main concern is infertility. In terms of reproduction, women with PCOS also have a greater risk for developing gestational diabetes (Joham et al. 2014). Inositols in the treatment and prevention of gestational diabetes is comprehensively discussed elsewhere in this book, but it is presumed that treatment with DCI may exert beneficial effects. Notably, women with PCOS are also at greater risk for metabolic syndrome and cardiovascular disease. Due to the increased metabolic risks associated with PCOS, further studies are needed using DCI alone, or in combination with MI, that are specifically focused on metabolic parameters, so that more definitive conclusions on metabolic outcomes of interest can be drawn.

While metformin is the preferred insulin sensitizer for the treatment of PCOS, the use of metformin may be limited by its gastrointestinal side effects. In contrast, the inositols are well tolerated with minimal to no side effects. In addition, not all women with PCOS respond satisfactorily to treatment with metformin. Therefore, in our opinion, MI+DCI combination therapy should be considered in women with PCOS who are unable to tolerate metformin or fail to respond adequately to metformin. Whether treatment with inositols in combination with metformin would offer benefits above those of treatment with metformin or inositols alone is unknown. Future, well-designed studies evaluating the effects of combination MI+DCI versus metformin, as well as the effects of all three treatments in combination, would help further elucidate treatment options for women with PCOS.

In summary, we found that currently available data is limited by small sample sizes, limited treatment durations, differences in outcome measures, inconsistency in dosing, incomplete publication of results and statistical testing, and the limited number of randomized placebo-controlled studies. Nonetheless, the results of basic science studies and subsequent small clinical trials collectively suggest that inositols are promising agents for the treatment of PCOS that merit further study and should be considered for the treatment of infertility in select women with PCOS as adjunctive therapy.

References

Artini, P. G., E. Casarosa, E. Carletti, P. Monteleone, A. Di Noia, and O. M. Di Berardino. 2017. "In vitro effect of myo-inositol on sperm motility in normal and oligoasthenospermia patients undergoing in vitro fertilization." *Gynecol Endocrinol* 33 (2):109-112. doi: 10.1080/09513590.2016.1254179.

Asplin, I., G. Galasko, and J. Larner. 1993. "chiro-inositol deficiency and insulin resistance: a comparison of the chiro-inositol- and the myo-inositol-containing insulin mediators isolated from urine, hemodialysate, and muscle of control and type II diabetic subjects." *Proc Natl Acad Sci US* 90 (13):5924-8.

Azziz, R., E. Carmina, D. Dewailly, E. Diamanti-Kandarakis, H. F. Escobar-Morreale, W. Futterweit, O. E. Janssen, R. S. Legro, R. J. Norman, A. E. Taylor, and S. F. Witchel. 2009. "The Androgen Excess and PCOS Society criteria for the polycystic ovary syndrome: the complete task force report." *Fertil Steril* 91 (2):456-88. doi: 10.1016/j.fertnstert.2008.06.035.

Baillargeon, J. P., M. J. Iuorno, D. J. Jakubowicz, T. Apridonidze, N. He, and J. E. Nestler. 2004. "Metformin Therapy Increases Insulin-Stimulated Release of d-Chiro-Inositol-Containing Inositolphosphoglycan Mediator in Women with Polycystic Ovary Syndrome." *The Journal of Clinical Endocrinology & Metabolism* 89 (1):242-249. doi: 10.1210/jc.2003-030437.

Benelli, E., S. Del Ghianda, C. Di Cosmo, and M. Tonacchera. 2016. *A Combined Therapy with Myo-Inositol and D-Chiro-Inositol Improves Endocrine Parameters and Insulin Resistance in PCOS Young Overweight Women*. Vol. 2016.

Birdsall, M. A., C. M. Farquhar, and H. D. White. 1997. "ASsociation between polycystic ovaries and extent of coronary artery disease in women having cardiac catheterization." *Annals of Internal Medicine* 126 (1):32-35. doi: 10.7326/0003-4819-126-1-199701010-00005.

Chiu, T. T., M. S. Rogers, E. L. Law, C. M. Briton-Jones, L. P. Cheung, and C. J. Haines. 2002. "Follicular fluid and serum concentrations of myo-inositol in patients undergoing IVF: relationship with oocyte quality." *Hum Reprod* 17 (6):1591-6.

Colazingari, S., M. Treglia, R. Najjar, and A. Bevilacqua. 2013. *The combined therapy myo-inositol plus D-chiro-inositol, rather than D-chiro-inositol, is able to improve IVF outcomes: Results from a randomized controlled trial.* Vol. 288.

Costantino, D., G. Minozzi, E. Minozzi, and C. Guaraldi. 2009. "Metabolic and hormonal effects of myo-inositol in women with polycystic ovary syndrome: a double-blind trial." *Eur Rev Med Pharmacol Sci* 13 (2):105-10.

Diamanti-Kandarakis, E., C. Kouli, T. Tsianateli, and A. Bergiele. 1998. "Therapeutic effects of metformin on insulin resistance and hyperandrogenism in polycystic ovary syndrome." *Eur J Endocrinol* 138 (3):269-74.

Dunaif, A., Karen Segal, Walter Futterweit, and A. Dobrjansky. 1989. *Profound Peripheral Insulin Resistance, Independent of Obesity, in Polycystic Ovary Syndrome*. Vol. 38.

Fruzzetti, F., Perini, D., Russo, M., Bucci, F., Gadduci, A. 2016. "Comparison of two insulin sensitizers, metformin and myo-inositol, in women with polycystic ovary syndrome (PCOS)." *Gynecological Endocrinology*, 33:1, 39-42, DOI: 10.1080/09513590.2016.1236078.

Foroozanfard, F., M. Samimi, K. H. Almadani, and M. Sehat. 2017. "Effect of metformin on the anti-Mullerian hormone level in infertile women with polycystic ovarian syndrome." *Electron Physician* 9 (12):5969-5973. doi: 10.19082/5969.

Genazzani, A. D., C. Lanzoni, F. Ricchieri, and V. M. Jasonni. 2008. "Myo-inositol administration positively affects hyperinsulinemia and hormonal parameters in overweight patients with polycystic ovary syndrome." *Gynecol Endocrinol* 24 (3):139-44. doi: 10.1080/095135 90801893232.

Gerli, S., E. Papaleo, A. Ferrari, and G. C. Di Renzo. 2007. "Randomized, double blind placebo-controlled trial: effects of myo-inositol on ovarian function and metabolic factors in women with PCOS." *Eur Rev Med Pharmacol Sci* 11 (5):347-54.

Heimark, D., J. McAllister, and J. Larner. 2014. "Decreased myo-inositol to chiro-inositol (M/C) ratios and increased M/C epimerase activity in PCOS theca cells demonstrate increased insulin sensitivity compared to controls." *Endocr J* 61 (2):111-7.

Isabella, R., and E. Raffone. 2012. "Does ovary need D-chiro-inositol?" *J Ovarian Res* 5 (1):14. doi: 10.1186/1757-2215-5-14.

Iuorno, M. J., D. J. Jakubowicz, J. P. Baillargeon, P. Dillon, R. D. Gunn, G. Allan, and J. E. Nestler. 2002. "Effects of d-chiro-inositol in lean women with the polycystic ovary syndrome." *Endocr Pract* 8 (6):417-23. doi: 10.4158/ep.8.6.417.

Jamilian M, Farhat P, Foroozanfard F, et al. Comparison of myo- inositol and metformin on clinical, metabolic and genetic parameters in polycystic ovary syndrome: A randomized controlled clinical trial. *Clin Endocrinol (Oxf).* 2017;87:194–200. https://doi.org/10.1111/cen.1336.

Jamilian M, Farhat P, Foroozanfard F, et al. Comparison of myo- inositol and metformin on clinical, metabolic and genetic parameters in polycystic ovary syndrome: A randomized controlled clinical trial. *Clin Endocrinol (Oxf).* 2017;87:194–200. https://doi.org/10.1111/cen.1336.

Jamilian M, Farhat P, Foroozanfard F, et al. 2017. "Comparison of myo-inositol and metformin on clinical, metabolic and genetic parameters in polycystic ovary syndrome: A randomized controlled clinical trial." *Clin Endocrinol (Oxf).* 87:194–200. https://doi.org/10.1111/cen.1336.

Joham, A. E., S. Ranasinha, S. Zoungas, L. Moran, and H. J. Teede. 2014. "Gestational Diabetes and Type 2 Diabetes in Reproductive-Aged Women with Polycystic Ovary Syndrome." *The Journal of Clinical Endocrinology & Metabolism* 99 (3):E447-E452. doi: 10.1210/jc.2013-2007.

Kennington, A. S., C. R. Hill, J. Craig, C. Bogardus, I. Raz, H. K. Ortmeyer, B. C. Hansen, G. Romero, and J. Larner. 1990. "Low Urinary chiro-Inositol Excretion in Non-Insulin-Dependent Diabetes Mellitus."

New England Journal of Medicine 323 (6):373-378. doi: 10.1056/NEJM199008093230603.

Knochenhauer, E. S., Key, T. J., Kahsar-Miller, M., Waggoner, W., Boots, L. R., Azziz, R. 1998. "Prevalence of polycystic ovary syndrome in unselected black and white women of the southeastern united states: a prospective study." *The Journal of Clinical Endocrinology & Metabolism*, 83(9); 3078-3082. DOI:10.1210/jcem.83.9.5090.

Larner, J. 2002. "D-chiro-inositol--its functional role in insulin action and its deficit in insulin resistance." *Int J Exp Diabetes Res* 3 (1):47-60.

Legro, R. S., A. R. Kunselman, W. C. Dodson, and A. Dunaif. 1999. "Prevalence and Predictors of Risk for Type 2 Diabetes Mellitus and Impaired Glucose Tolerance in Polycystic Ovary Syndrome: A Prospective, Controlled Study in 254 Affected Women1." *The Journal of Clinical Endocrinology & Metabolism* 84 (1):165-169. doi: 10.1210/jcem.84.1.5393.

Mani, H., Levy. M. J., Davies. M. J., D. H. Morris, L. J. Gray, J. Bankart, H. Blackledge, K. Khunti, and T. A. Howlett. 2012. "Diabetes and cardiovascular events in women with polycystic ovary syndrome: a 20-year retrospective cohort study." *Clinical Endocrinology* 78 (6):926-934. doi: 10.1111/cen.12068.

Minozzi, M., M. Nordio, and R. Pajalich. 2013. "The Combined therapy myo-inositol plus D-Chiro-inositol, in a physiological ratio, reduces the cardiovascular risk by improving the lipid profile in PCOS patients." *Eur Rev Med Pharmacol Sci* 17 (4):537-40.

Nestler, J. E., D. J. Jakubowicz, P. Reamer, R. D. Gunn, and G. Allan. 1999. "Ovulatory and metabolic effects of D-chiro-inositol in the polycystic ovary syndrome." *N Engl J Med* 340 (17):1314-20. doi: 10.1056/nejm199904293401703.

Nestler, J. E., G. Romero, L. C. Huang, C. G. Zhang, and J. Larner. 1991. "Insulin mediators are the signal transduction system responsible for insulin's actions on human placental steroidogenesis." *Endocrinology* 129 (6):2951-6. doi: 10.1210/endo-129-6-2951.

Nestler, J. E. 2008. "Metformin for the treatment of polycystic ovary syndrome." *N Engl J Med* 358:47-54. DOI: 10.1056/NEJMct0707092.

Nordio, M., and E. Proietti. 2012. "The combined therapy with myo-inositol and D-chiro-inositol reduces the risk of metabolic disease in PCOS overweight patients compared to myo-inositol supplementation alone." *Eur Rev Med Pharmacol Sci* 16 (5):575-81.

Orio, F., Jr., S. Palomba, T. Cascella, B. De Simone, S. Di Biase, T. Russo, D. Labella, F. Zullo, G. Lombardi, and A. Colao. 2004. "Early impairment of endothelial structure and function in young normal-weight women with polycystic ovary syndrome." *J Clin Endocrinol Metab* 89 (9):4588-93. doi: 10.1210/jc.2003-031867.

Papaleo, E., V. Unfer, J. P. Baillargeon, F. Fusi, F. Occhi, and L. De Santis. 2009. "Myo-inositol may improve oocyte quality in intracytoplasmic sperm injection cycles. A prospective, controlled, randomized trial." *Fertil Steril* 91 (5):1750-4. doi: 10.1016/j.fertnstert.2008.01.088.

Penzias, A., Bendikson, K., Butts, S., Coutifaris, C., Falcone, T., Fossum, G., Gitlin, S., Gracia, C., Hansen, K., La Barbera, A., Mersereau, J., Odem, R., Paulson, R., Pfeifer, S., Pisarska, M., Rebar, R., Reindollar, R., Rosen, M., Sandlow, J., Vernon, M., Practice Committee of the American Society for Reproductive Medicine. 2017. "Role of metformin for ovulation induction in infertile patients with polycystic ovary syndrome (PCOS): a guideline." *Fertil Steril* 108 (3):426-441. doi: 10.1016/j.fertnstert.2017.06.026.

Raffone, E., P. Rizzo, and V. Benedetto. 2010. "Insulin sensitiser agents alone and in co-treatment with r-FSH for ovulation induction in PCOS women." *Gynecol Endocrinol* 26 (4):275-80. doi: 10.3109/095135 90903366996.

Rotterdam, ESHRE/ASRM-Sponsored PCOS Consensus Workshop Group. 2004. "Revised 2003 consensus on diagnostic criteria and long-term health risks related to polycystic ovary syndrome." *Fertil Steril* 81 (1):19-25.

Sharma, S. T., E. P. Wickham, 3rd, and J. E. Nestler. 2007. "Changes in glucose tolerance with metformin treatment in polycystic ovary syndrome: a retrospective analysis." *Endocr Pract* 13 (4):373-9. doi: 10.4158/ep.13.4.373.

Solomon, C. G., F. B. Hu, A. Dunaif, J. E. Rich-Edwards, M. J. Stampfer, W. C. Willett, F. E. Speizer, and J. E. Manson. 2002. "Menstrual cycle irregularity and risk for future cardiovascular disease." *J Clin Endocrinol Metab* 87 (5):2013-7. doi: 10.1210/jcem.87.5.8471.

Stein, I. F., and M. L. Leventhal. 1935. "Amenorrhea associated with bilateral polycystic ovaries." *American Journal of Obstetrics & Gynecology* 29 (2):181-191. doi: 10.1016/S0002-9378(15)30642-6.

Tagliaferri, V., Romualdi, D., Immediata, V., De Cicco, S., Di Florio C., Lanzone, A., Guido, M. "Metformin versus myoinositol: which is better in obese PCOS patients? A randomized controlled crossover study." *Clinical Endocrinology* 86, 725-730.

Unfer, V., G. Carlomagno, E. Papaleo, S. Vailati, M. Candiani, and J. P. Baillargeon. 2014. "Hyperinsulinemia Alters Myoinositol to d-chiroinositol Ratio in the Follicular Fluid of Patients with PCOS." *Reprod Sci* 21 (7):854-858. doi: 10.1177/1933719113518985.

Unfer, V., Facchinetti, F., Orru, B., Giordani B., Nestler, J., 2017. "Myo-inositol effects in women with PCOS: a meta-anlaysis of randomized controlled trials." *Endocrine Connections* 6, 647-658. doi:10.1530/EC-17-0243.

Willis, D., and S. Franks. 1995. "Insulin action in human granulosa cells from normal and polycystic ovaries is mediated by the insulin receptor and not the type-I insulin-like growth factor receptor." *J Clin Endocrinol Metab* 80 (12):3788-90. doi: 10.1210/jcem.80.12.8530637.

Zawadzki, J. K. 1992. "Diagnostic Criteria for Polycystic Ovary Syndrome: Towards a Rational Approach." *NIH Expert Conference on PCOS*.

In: Inositols
Editor: Vittorio Unfer
ISBN: 978-1-53614-912-8

Chapter 4

INOSITOLS AND METABOLIC SYNDROME

Marine L. Croze*[1]*, PhD
and Christophe O. Soulage*[2,*]*, PhD
[1]Montreal Diabetes Research Center
and Research Center of the Montreal University Hospital Center,
Montreal University, Montreal, Quebec, Canada
[2]Univ. Lyon, INSA de Lyon,
Université Claude Bernard Lyon 1, Villeurbanne, France

ABSTRACT

There is accumulating evidence that some inositol isomers, especially myo-inositol and D-chiro-inositol, could be beneficial in the prevention and/or the treatment of insulin resistance states. Some inositol isomers or derivatives exhibit potent insulin-mimetic or insulin sensitizing actions and efficiently lower blood glucose levels. Thus, the aim of this review is to provide current evidence on the potential benefits of inositols in the management of pathologic states associated with insulin resistance such as metabolic syndrome, gestational diabetes or type 2 diabetes.

---

* Corresponding Author's Email: christophe.soulage@insa-lyon.fr.

Keywords: inositols, insulin resistance, metabolic syndrome, diabetes, gestational diabetes

INTRODUCTION

The metabolic syndrome is classically defined as a set of clinical features (Reaven 2006), most of them being related to insulin resistance, including some of the following: abdominal obesity, hyperinsulinemia, impaired glucose tolerance, increased plasma triglycerides, decreased HDL cholesterol and hypertension. Often, metabolic syndrome is the first step in the development of type 2 diabetes (T2D). Insulin resistance is a pathological condition in which cells and tissues (especially skeletal muscle, white adipose tissue and liver) fail to respond normally to insulin (Petersen and Shulman 2006; Samuel and Shulman 2012). Insulin resistance impairs the metabolic homeostasis and triggers many deleterious effects. When cells and tissues become insulin resistant, the uptake of glucose into muscle and adipose cells is blunted, promoting hyperglycemia; Hyperglycemia is compensated by an exaggerated secretion of insulin (i.e., hyperinsulinemia) that in turn promotes lipid and cholesterol synthesis and storage. Since glucose uptake is deficient in muscle and adipose tissue, more glucose is directed to the liver where it is converted and stored into the form of triglycerides (e.g., fatty liver). Blood triglycerides and non esterified fatty acids are raised leading to ectopic lipid storage in muscle and liver. Ectopic lipid redistribution leads to lipotoxicity that further impair insulin signaling.

To date, several insulin sensitizing drugs have been used to alleviate insulin resistance amongst which some inositols and inositol derivatives (Croze and Soulage 2013; Muscogiuri et al. 2016; Joseph Larner, Brautigan, and Thorner 2010; Joseph Larner 2002; J. Larner 2001). Inositols are polyols naturally occuring in animals and plants, either in their free forms or as constitutents of phospholipids or inositol phosphate derivatives. Inositol exists under nine stereoisomeric forms depending on the spatial orientation of its six hydroxyl groups (Figure 1). Inositols are involved in many key

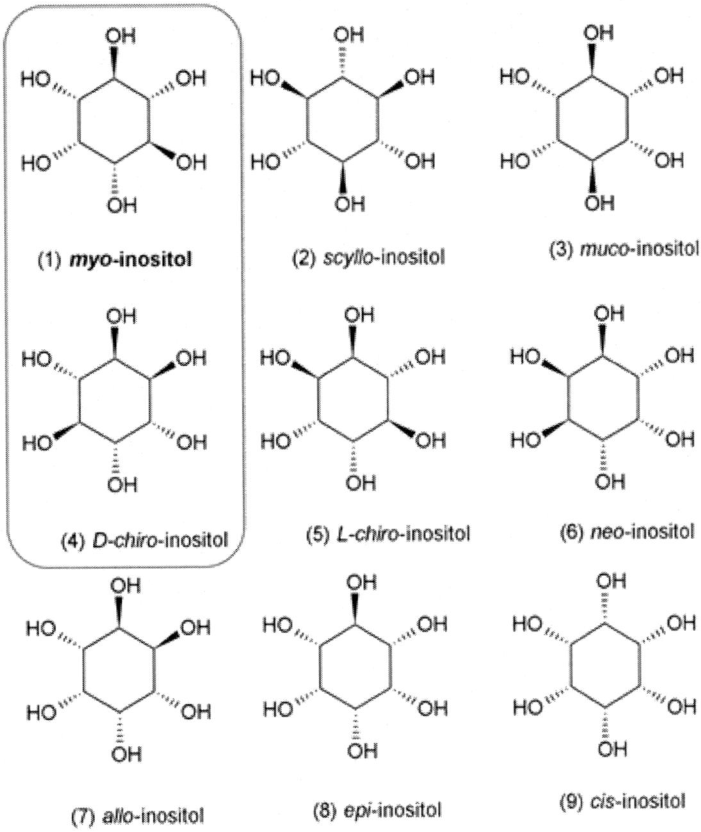

Figure 1. Structures of the nine stereoisomers of inositol. Myo-inositol and D-chiro-inositol (both framed) are the most common isomers of inositol used in experimental and clinical studies. Note that myo-inositol is the most common isomer of inositol in foodstuffs and animal tissues.

cellular processes, as the structural basis for secondary messengers in eukaryotic cells, and in particular as inositol triphosphates (IP_3), phosphatidyl inositol phosphate lipids (PIP_2/PIP_3) and inositol glycans, described as putative mediators of the insulin signaling pathway. Recent experimental and clinical evidences suggest that supplementation with inositols (myo-inositol, D-chiro-inositol, D-pinitol) as a dietary supplement could be beneficial in various pathological states, particularly those associated with glucose intolerance and insulin resistance. Thus, the aim of this review is to provide current evidence[1] on the potential benefits of inositol isomers or derivatives in the management of pathologic states associated with insulin resistance. These conditions include metabolic syndrome, pre-diabetes, gestational diabetes mellitus and polycystic ovary syndrome (PCOS).

Benefits of Inositols in Preclinical Models of Metabolic Diseases

There is some evidences about the beneficial effects of some inositols or inositol derivatives on glucose metabolism in a large range of species and animal models of metabolic diseases (for instance rats treated with streptozotocin (Bates, Jones, and Bailey 2000), obese ob/ob mice (Bates, Jones, and Bailey 2000; Shen et al. 2012), diabetic Rhesus monkey (Ortmeyer, Bodkin, et al. 1993; Ortmeyer, Huang, et al. 1993) and so on…). Four compounds were extensively studied: myo-inositol (MI), D-chiro-inositol (DCI), sequoyitol and D-pinitol.

Myo-Inositol

The blood glucose lowering action of dietary MI was historically demonstrated in type 2 diabetic Rhesus monkey (Ortmeyer, Bodkin, et al. 1993; Ortmeyer, Huang, et al. 1993). MI was proved to improve glucose tolerance in control mice. This effect was associated with an improvement in peripheral insulin sensitivity as evidenced by an increased GLUT-4 translocation to the plasma membrane in the skeletal muscle (Dang et al. 2010; Croze et al. 2013). MI (associated to Vitamins B and D) improved insulin sensitivity in a mouse model of gestational diabetes i.e., dams of db/+

[1] Methodology: We searched in the Medline® database (using PubMed as a search engine) with the thesaurus term "INOSITOL" combined using the Boolean operator "AND" with the thesaurus terms "METABOLIC SYNDROME", "INSULIN RESISTANCE" or "DIABETES MELLITUS". Papers were restricted to those published in English.

mice (Plows et al. 2017). Dietary supplementation with MI in diabetic rat dams is associated with an increase in tissue MI levels and a decrease in foetal malformations suggesting it could be used to prevent diabetic embryopathy (Khandelwal et al. 1998; Reece et al. 1997)[2]. MI inhibits intestinal glucose absorption and increases muscle glucose uptake (in presence as well as in absence of insulin) (Chukwuma, Ibrahim, and Islam 2016). MI (25 and 50 mg/kg/day) improved glyceamic control and dyslipidemia in rat injected with streptozotocin and fed a high-fat diet (Antony et al. 2017) by improving insulin signaling. In Human Umbillical Vein Endothelial Cells (HUVEC) MI (as well as DCI) acts as an insulin mimetic drug and stimulates phosphorylation of protein kinase/Akt more efficiently than insulin (D'Oria et al. 2017). Some other studies however yielded conflicting results. In one study, in rat with streptozotocin induced diabetes, MI failed to improve glyceamic control (Greene, De Jesus, and Winegrad 1975) while it prevented diabetic neuropathy. Dietary MI supplementation was efficient in the prevention of inositol intra-tissue depletion, but did not prevent insulin resistance associated with obesity in mice fed an high fat diet (Croze, Géloën, and Soulage 2015). The large differences in animal models and experimental settings could account for these discrepancies.

D-Chiro-Inositol

DCI was also proved to act as an insulin mimetic and insulin sensitizing compound (Joseph Larner 2002; J. Larner 2001; Asplin, Galasko, and Larner 1993). DCI glycans normalize plasma glucose in streptozotocin diabetic rats as efficiently as insulin without inducing any hypoglycaemia (Fonteles, Huang, and Larner 1996). Associated with manganese chloride (8.3μg/kg), DCI (15 mg/kg) decreased plasma glucose in low dose streptozotocin-treated rats (Fonteles, Almeida, and Larner 2000). DCI (30-60 mg/kg/day) improved insulin-mediated glucose uptake through stimulation of the

---

[2] A recent meta-analysis on the effect of MI intake in women at risk of gestational diabetes however challenged this view (Crawford et al. 2015).

Phosphatidyl inositol 3 kinase (PI3K)/Akt signaling pathway in rat model of T2D (Gao et al. 2016). Oral administration of DCI to diabetic KK-A(y) mice lowered plasma glucose, C-peptide, improved glucose tolerance, and increased insulin content in the pancreas (Yao et al. 2008). Streptozotocin-induced diabetic mice treated for 60 days with DCI (20 mg/kg, twice a day) exhibited an improvement of both autonomic and somatic neuropathy (Farias et al. 2011).

Sequoyitol (5-O-Methyl-Myo-Inositol)

The derivative of MI, 5-O-Methyl-myo-inositol, also referred to as sequoyitol, exerts potent anti-diabetic effects in mice. Indeed, administrations of sequoyitol (80mg/kg/day) for 8-10 weeks improved glycemic control and restored insulin signaling in the liver of ob/ob mice (Shen et al. 2012). Sequoyitol further ameliorates hyperglycemia and glucose intolerance by increasing both insulin sensitivity and insulin secretion (Shen et al. 2012). Sequoyitol prevented the progression of diabetic nephropathy in diabetic rats (induced by a high-fat diet and a low dose of streptozotocin) through its glucose-lowering effects, antioxidant activity, and regulation of Tissue Growth Factor Beta1(TGF-β_1) expression (Li et al. 2014).

D-Pinitol (3-O-Methyl-Chiroinositol)

D-pinitol was proved to be hepato- (Sivakumar, Palsamy, and Subramanian 2010a) and reno- protective (Sivakumar, Palsamy, and Subramanian 2010b) (through anti-inflammatory and antioxidant activities) in streptozotocin-induced diabetic rats. D-Pinitol further protects the pancreatic tissue from free radical-mediated oxidative stress (Sivakumar and Subramanian 2009). D-pinitol exhibited potent antihyperlipidemic effect in STZ-induced type 2 diabetic rats (Geethan and Prince 2008). D-pinitol exerts an insulin-like effect and improves glycaemic control in hypoinsulinaemic streptozotocin-diabetic mice (Bates, Jones, and Bailey 2000). D-pinitol at a bolus dose of 5 mg/kg decreased plasma glucose in low dose streptozotocin-treated rats (Fonteles, Almeida, and Larner 2000).

Inositol Glycans

Inositol phosphoglycans were described as putative second messengers of insulin action (Reddy, Falck, and Capdevila 1993; Plourde, D'Alarcao, and Saltiel 1992; Frick et al. 1998a, 1998b; Joseph Larner, Brautigan, and Thorner 2010). In vitro synthetized acylated inositol glycans (AIG) exhibit insulin-like activities and improve glucose tolerance in several mice models of diabetes with or without obesity (Suzuki et al. 2014). DCI glycan stimulates insulin secretion in pancreas β cells (Lazarenko et al. 2014). However, the exact structure-activity relationship of inositol phosphoglycans is not precisely defined and one study yielded conflicting results since over a wide range of synthetic inositol phosphoglycans, none were insulin mimetic (Hecht et al. 2010).

Benefits of Inositols in Patients with Insulin Resistance and Related Diseases

MI and D-chiro-inositol were shown to improve insulin sensitivity and ovulatory function in women with PCOS (Paul et al. 2016). The use of inositol in PCOS has revieved extensive attention. Metabolic effects of inositols in women with PCOS will not be discussed in the present review and are the subject of a specific chapter (Chapter 6). The main results of clinical studies with inositols or inositol derivatives in the context of metabolic diseases are summarized in Table 1.

Table 1. Clinical trials with inositol supplementation evaluated for the treatment or prevention of metabolic diseases

Reference	Study design	Duration	Treatment	Nb	Population	Results
Maurizi et al. 2017	Randomized, controlled vs. Placebo	24 weeks	1g DCI + 400 µg folic acid/day	N = 26 DCI: N = 13 Placebo: N = 11	Patients with T1D Males/Females: 13/13	Decrease in HbA1c level
Farren et al. 2017	Randomized, controlled vs. Placebo	24 to 28 weeks of gestation	1.1g MI +27.6 mg DCI + 400 µg folic acid /day	N = 240 MI+DCI: N = 120 Placebo: N = 120	Pregnant women with a family history of diabetes	No difference in the incidence of GDM
Bañul et al. 2016	Double-blind, randomized, controlled vs placebo	12 weeks	Inositol-enriched beverage (IEB): 2.23g twice a day	N = 44 Inositols: N = 24 Placebo: N = 20	Patients with impaired fasting glucose. Males/Females: 15/29	Decrease in insulin, HOMA-IR and percentage of glucose change after postprandial /fasting period
Lubin et al. 2016	Prospective study, not randomized, not controlled	12 months	1.2g MI + 400µg folic acid /day	N = 60 MI: N = 32 Insulin: N = 28	Women with GDM not controlled by the diet	No difference between groups Less labour induction in MI group. OR: 0.22 (95%CI 0.07–0.65)
Santamaria et al. 2016	Open label, randomized, controlled vs. Placebo	from the first trimester through the whole pregnancy	2g MI + 200µg folic acid twice a day	N = 197 MI: N = 95 Placebo: N = 102	Pregnant overweighted non-obese women	Decreased incidence of GDM OR 0.33 (95% CI 0.15–0.70)
D'Anna et al. 2013	Randomized, controlled vs. placebo, open-label	from the first trimester through the whole pregnancy	2g MI + 200 µg folic acid twice a day	N = 220 MI: N = 110 Placebo: N = 110	Pregnant women with family history of T2D	Decreased incidence of GDM OR 0.35 (95%CI, 0.13-0.96)
Matarrelli et al. 2013	randomized, controlled vs. placebo, double-blind	throughout pregnancy	4g MI + 400 µg folic acid/ day	N = 73 MI: N = 35 Placebo: N = 38	Non-obese pregnant women /elevated fasting glucose	Lower incidence of abnormal OGTT. RR, 0.127 (95% CI, 0.032–0.502)

Reference	Study design	Duration	Treatment	Nb	Population	Results
Santamaria et al. 2012	Randomized, controlled vs. placebo	12 months	MI 2g /day	N = 80 MI: N = 40 Placebo: N = 40	Postmenopausal women with MetS	Serum glucose, insulin, HOMA-IR, TG, total and HDL-cholesterol and BP significantly improved with MI
Kim et al. 2012	Randomized, double-blind, placebo-controlled	12 weeks	400 mg D-pinitol, three times a day	N = 66 D-pinitol: N = 33 Placebo: N = 33	Patients with T2D	Decrease in HbA1c, fasting plasma glucose, and HOMA-IR
Giordano et al. 2011	Randomized, controlled vs. placebo	6 months	MI 2g/day	N = 80 MI: N = 40 Placebo: N = 40	Postmenopausal women with MetS	Decrease in diastolic BP, HOMA-IR, serum TG. Increase in HDL cholesterol
Corrado et al. 2011	Randomized, controlled vs. placebo, open label	8 weeks	2g MI + 200µg folic acid, twice/day	N = 69 MI: N = 24 Placebo: N = 45	Women with GDM	Decreased glycaemia, insulinemia and HOMA-IR
Maeba et al. 2008	Not a placebo controlled study	2 weeks	5g MI/day the 1st week, 10g MI/day the 2nd week	N = 17	Hyperlipidemic subjects with or without MetS. Males/females: 15/2	Decrease in sdLDL
Kim et al. 2005	Randomized, double-blinded, placebo controlled	13 weeks	600 mg D-pinitol twice daily	N = 30 D-pinitol: N = 15 Placebo: N = 15	Patients with T2D. Males/Females: 14/16	Decrease in fasting plasma glucose, insulin, fructosamine, HbA1c, HOMA-IR, LDL-cholesterol and BP. Increase in HDL-cholesterol
Davis et al. 2000	Randomized, double-blinded, placebo controlled	28 days	20mg D-pinitol/kg/day	N = 22 D-pinitol: N = 12 Placebo: N = 10	Obese patients with mild type 2 diabetes. Males/Females: 12/10	HE clamp: No difference in baseline glucose production, insulin-mediated glucose disposal, or rates of appearance of free fatty acids

Abbreviations: BP, Blood Pressure; 95%CI, 95% Confidence Interval; DCI, D-chiroinositol; GDM, Gestational Diabetes Mellitus; HDL, High Density Lipoprotein; HE clamp, Hyperinsulinemic Euglycaemic clamp; HOMA-IR, HOmeostasis Model Assessment of Insulin Resistance; IEB, Inositol Enriched Beverage; LDL, Low Density Lipoprotein; MetS, Metabolic Syndrome; MI, myo-inositol; OGTT, Oral Glucose Tolerance Test; OR, Odd Ratio; RR, Relative Risk; sdLDL, small dense LDL; T1D, Type 1 Diabetes; T2D, Type 2 Diabetes; TG, triglycerides.

Inositols Supplementation in Women with Metabolic Syndrome or Gestational Diabetes

Daily supplementation with MI can prevent or improve insulin resistance in post-menopausal women with metabolic syndrome as well as in pregnant women at risk of gestational diabetes (D'Anna et al. 2013b; Matarrelli et al. 2013; Corrado et al. 2011; Angelo Santamaria et al. 2016; Giordano et al. 2011). A daily supplementation with 2g of MI for 8 weeks in women with gestational diabetes decreased fasting insulinemia and glycemia (-42% compared to the placebo group with diet modifications only) (Corrado et al. 2011). Similar benefits were observed in postmenopausal women with metabolic syndrome supplemented for 12 months with MI (2g/day) as evidenced by a significant decrease of the HOMA-IR (Homeostasis model assessment of insulin resistance[1]) index (-78% compared to the placebo group with the dietary intervention only) (A. Santamaria et al. 2012). Interestingly in postmenopausal women, the cardiovascular risk parameters were also further improved with the MI supplement with a reduction in blood pressure, in LDL-cholesterol, in serum triglycerides (-34%) and an increase in HDL-cholesterol (+21%). At the end of the study, 8 women out of 40 in the MI group (i.e., 20%) did not exhibit anymore a metabolic syndrome compared to only one out of the 40 patients (i.e., 2.5%) in the placebo group with the diet alone. The most important result of Santamaria et al. study is the critical reduction in insulinemia and insulin resistance (estimated through HOMA-IR), which was greater than with other insulin-sensitizing substances such as pioglitazone (Gupta et al. 2009a), rosiglitazone (Esposito et al. 2006a) and metformin (Fontbonne et al. 2009a), considered as golden standards in patients with impaired glucose tolerance. MI was more effective than rosiglitazone (Esposito et al. 2006b) in reducing serum triglycerides although less effective than pioglitazone (Gupta et al. 2009a) (i.e., -50%, -34% and -20% for rosiglitazone, MI and pioglitazone, respectively) (Esposito et al. 2006a). Thus MI supplementation

---

[1] HOMA-IR, a common index of insulin resistance, is calculated as Fasting insulin (mIU/L) x Fasting glucose (mg/dL) / 405 or Fasting insulin (mIU/L) x Fasting glucose (mmol/L) / 22.5.

could be an effective treatment to reduce cardiovascular risk profile in a context of metabolic syndrome. In pregnant women with a family history of T2D, MI (given at 4g/day throughout the pregnancy) also significantly improved the glucose tolerance during an hyperglycemic challenge, and significantly reduced the incidence of gestational diabetes (OR 0.35 95%CI: 0.13-0.96) (D'Anna et al. 2013a). The supplementation of pregnant women with MI further reduced some hyperglycemia-related fetal outcomes, such as fetal macrosomia and high birth weight. Women with gestational diabetes insufficiently controlled by diet (n = 32) were successfully treated with MI 1.2g/day and folic acid 400µg/day for 12 months (Lubin et al. 2016) suggesting that MI could be a safe first-line therapy for gestational diabetes that is not controlled by lifestyle changes. MI (4g MI +400 µg folic acid per day, throughout pregnancy) improved insulin resistance and reduced the incidence of abnormal OGTT (RR, 0.127, 95% CI: 0.032–0.502) in women at risk of gestational diabetes (Matarrelli, Vitacolonna, D'Angelo, et al. 2013). Eighty postmenopausal women with metabolic syndrome were treated with a low-energy diet, and MI (2 g/day) for 12 months. At the end of the study, women with MI exhibited a significant improvement of HOMA-IR and blood lipids compared to the placebo group (A. Santamaria et al. 2012). The incidence of gestational diabetes was significantly lower in the MI group compared to the placebo group (11.6% versus 27.4%, respectively). In a recent randomized clinical trial, including 240 women with a familly history of T2D, Farren et al. however failed to show any benefits of a combination of MI (1,100 mg/day) and DCI (27.6 mg/day) in early pregnancy (24 to 28 weeks of gestation) to prevent gestational diabetes (Farren et al. 2017); however needs to be noticed that in this study important factors were not considered in order to extrapolate univocal results. First, women with a family history in a first-degree relative of diabetes, either type 1 diabetes (T1D) or T2D, were included. With T1D relatives there might be different genetic predisposition to develop GDM in respect to T2D. Furthermore, selection of the study population was wide, including diverse risk factors for GDM, such as obesity and previous GDM. This was well discussed in a letter by Pintaudi and Di Vieste (2017), which carefully reviewed the study design and found various important criticism.

In a randomized clinical trial, MI (2 g plus 200 μg folic acid twice a day) or placebo (200 μg folic acid twice a day) was administered from the first trimester to delivery in pregnant overweight non-obese women (Angelo Santamaria et al. 2016). MI treatment was associated with a 67% reduction in the incidence of gestational diabetes (OR 0.33; 95% CI, 0.15–0.70). Several randomized controlled trials (D'Anna et al. 2013b; D'Anna et al. 2015; Angelo Santamaria et al. 2016) and two meta-analyses demonstrated the beneficial effects of MI dietary supplementation. Zheng et al. (Zheng et al. 2015) demonstrated that supplementation with MI was associated with a significant reduction in the incidence of gestational diabetes (RR, 0.29; 95% CI: 0.19-0.44, 5 trials, n = 513 women). In the Cochrane database meta analysis (Crawford et al. 2015), the supplementation with MI was associated with a reduction in the incidence of gestational diabetes compared with control (RR 0.43, 95% CI: 0.29 -0.64; 3 trials; n = 502 women). However, two major limits were pinpointed by these authors: i) All of the studies included in the latter metaanalysis were conducted in Italy which raises concerns about generalisability of the results of the study to other settings. ii) the quality of the evidences were of low or very low quality. Furthermore, one should keep in mind that all these studies only included women with a special hormonal status (gestation, post-menopause,...) which do not enable us to conclude on the effect of MI supplementation in the general context of metabolic syndrome. Additional studies on larger populations, from different origins, sex and in double-blind trials should be done to unambiguously demonstrate the potency of inositols supplementation as an insulin-sensitizing treatment.

Inositols Supplementation in Patients with Prediabetes or T2D

The DCI and MI concentrations are increased in the urine of T2D patients and the urinary product (i.e., DCI concentration multiplied by MI concentration) is a potent biomarker of T2D (Hong et al. 2012). A diagnostic toolkit for the measurement of urinary myo-inositol (Lucica MI) had been developed (based on an enzymatic assay) to detect glucose intolerance and diabetes mellitus at an early stage in disease progression. Clinical trial results demonstrated that the test could be used not only to detect diabetes mellitus, but also to predict impaired glucose tolerance at early stages (Yamakoshi and Kawazu 2008). DCI (associated with folic acid) improved metabolic control in overweighted T1D patients as evidenced by a significant decrease in HbA1c levels (7.5% versus 7.9% in patients supplemented with MI and controls, respectively) (Maurizi et al. 2017). Daily consumption of inositol-enriched beverage (containing mainly D-pinitol, 2g, twice a day for 12 weeks) in prediabetic subjects alleviated insulin resistance and improved postprandial glycemia in non-obese subjects while it decreased inflammation in obese subjects (Bañuls et al. 2016). A single dose of soybean-derived D-pinitol (0.6 g, 60 min before a meal) improved postprandial glycemia in patients with T2D (Kang et al. 2006). D-pinitol (1.2g/day for 3 months) improves glycemic control and insulin sensitivity in patients with T2D mellitus. D-pinitol was even more effective in patients with insulin resistance as evidenced by the higher HOMA-IR index (H. J. Kim et al. 2012). The same team demonstrated that D-pinitol treatment (20 mg/kg/day for 12-week) improved fasting glucose, post-prandial glucose levels, and HbA1c in T2D patients (H. J. Kim et al. 2012). Soybean-derived D-pinitol (0.6g, twice daily) was administered to Korean patients with T2D for 13 weeks (J.-I. Kim et al. 2005). D-pinitol significantly improved insulin sensitivity (estimated by a decrease in HOMA-IR) and decreased total cholesterol, LDL-cholesterol, LDL/HDL-cholesterol ratio, blood pressure and increased HDL-cholesterol. Taken together, these data suggest that D-pinitol may be beneficial in reducing cardiovascular risk in patient with T2D. These works on D-pinitol have however several limits: 1- All the clinical studies were performed by the same investigators. 2- All of these studies were conducted in Korea which raises concerns about generalisability of the results of the study to other settings. 3- These randomized clinical trials only included a limited number of patients (~30 patients in each arm). In contrast, in a very small study (10-12 patients per arm) D-pinitol (20mg/kg/day), demonstrated that four weeks of supplementation with D-pinitol did not improve insulin sensitivity in patients with obesity and mild T2D (Davis et al. 2000). MI treatment increases serum plasmalogens and decreases small dense LDL in hyperlipidemic subjects with metabolic syndrome (Maeba et al. 2008).

Conclusion

Evidence from the different trials of dietary supplementation with inositols in pathological states associated with insulin resistance (metabolic syndrome, post-menopausal women, gestational diabetes, etc.) showed a potential benefit. However, the current evidences are mainly based on monocentric, small-sized trials and in specific populations that raises some concerns about the lack of generalisability of these evidences. Further randomized controlled trials with inositols are encouraged and should include different ethnicities and varying risk factors.

Conflict of Interest

None.

References

Antony, P. J., G. R. Gandhi, A. Stalin, K. Balakrishna, E. Toppo, K. Sivasankaran, S. Ignacimuthu, and N. A. Al-Dhabi. 2017. Myoinositol Ameliorates High-Fat Diet and Streptozotocin-Induced Diabetes in Rats through Promoting Insulin Receptor Signaling. *Biomedicine & Pharmacotherapy = Biomedecine & Pharmacotherapie* 88 (avril): 1098 -1113. https://doi.org/10.1016/j.biopha.2017.01.170.

Asplin, I., G. Galasko, and J. Larner. 1993. Chiro-Inositol Deficiency and Insulin Resistance: A Comparison of the Chiro-Inositol- and the Myo-Inositol-Containing Insulin Mediators Isolated from Urine, Hemodialysate, and Muscle of Control and Type II Diabetic Subjects.

Proceedings of the National Academy of Sciences of the United States of America 90 (13): 5924‐28.

Bañuls, C., S. Rovira-Llopis, S. López-Doménech, S. Veses, V. M. Víctor, M. Rocha, and A. Hernández-Mijares. 2016. Effect of Consumption of a Carob Pod Inositol-Enriched Beverage on Insulin Sensitivity and Inflammation in Middle-Aged Prediabetic Subjects. *Food & Function* 7 (10): 4379‐87. https://doi.org/10.1039/c6fo01021k.

Bates, S. H., R. B. Jones, and C. J. Bailey. 2000. Insulin-like Effect of Pinitol. *British Journal of Pharmacology* 130 (8): 1944‐48. https://doi.org/10.1038/sj.bjp.0703523.

Chukwuma, C. I., M. A. Ibrahim, and Md S. Islam. 2016. Myo-Inositol Inhibits Intestinal Glucose Absorption and Promotes Muscle Glucose Uptake: A Dual Approach Study. *Journal of Physiology and Biochemistry* 72 (4): 791‐801. https://doi.org/10.1007/s13105-016-0517-1.

Corrado, F., R. D’Anna, G. Di Vieste, D. Giordano, B. Pintaudi, A. Santamaria, and A. Di Benedetto. 2011. The Effect of Myoinositol Supplementation on Insulin Resistance in Patients with Gestational Diabetes. *Diabetic Medicine: A Journal of the British Diabetic Association* 28 (8): 972‐75. https://doi.org/10.1111/j.1464-5491.2011.03284.x.

Crawford, Tineke J., Caroline A. Crowther, J. Alsweiler, and J. Brown. 2015. Antenatal Dietary Supplementation with Myo-Inositol in Women during Pregnancy for Preventing Gestational Diabetes. *The Cochrane Database of Systematic Reviews*, n° 12 (décembre): CD011507. https://doi.org/10.1002/14651858.CD011507.pub2.

Croze, M. L., A. Géloën, and C. O. Soulage. 2015. Abnormalities in Myo-Inositol Metabolism Associated with Type 2 Diabetes in Mice Fed a High-Fat Diet: Benefits of a Dietary Myo-Inositol Supplementation. *The British Journal of Nutrition* 113 (12): 1862‐75. https://doi.org/10.1017/S000711451500121X.

Croze, M. L., and C. O. Soulage. 2013. Potential Role and Therapeutic Interests of Myo-Inositol in Metabolic Diseases. *Biochimie* 95 (10): 1811‑27. https://doi.org/10.1016/j.biochi.2013.05.011.

Croze, M. L., R. E. Vella, N. J. Pillon, H. A. Soula, L. Hadji, M. Guichardant, and C. O. Soulage. 2013. Chronic Treatment with Myo-Inositol Reduces White Adipose Tissue Accretion and Improves Insulin Sensitivity in Female Mice. *The Journal of Nutritional Biochemistry* 24 (2): 457‑66. https://doi.org/10.1016/j.jnutbio.2012.01.008.

Dang, N. T., R. Mukai, K. I.Yoshida, and H. Ashida. 2010. D-Pinitol and Myo-Inositol Stimulate Translocation of Glucose Transporter 4 in Skeletal Muscle of C57BL/6 Mice. *Bioscience, Biotechnology, and Biochemistry* 74 (5): 1062‑67. https://doi.org/10.1271/bbb.90963.

D'Anna, R., A. Di Benedetto, A. Scilipoti, A. Santamaria, M. L. Interdonato, E. Petrella, I. Neri, B. Pintaudi, F. Corrado, and F. Facchinetti. 2015. Myo-Inositol Supplementation for Prevention of Gestational Diabetes in Obese Pregnant Women: A Randomized Controlled Trial. *Obstetrics and Gynecology* 126 (2): 310‑15. https://doi.org/10.1097/AOG.0000000000000958.

D'Anna, R., A. Scilipoti, D. Giordano, C. Caruso, M. L. Cannata, M. L. Interdonato, F. Corrado, and A. Di Benedetto. 2013a. Myo-Inositol Supplementation and Onset of Gestational Diabetes Mellitus in Pregnant Women With a Family History of Type 2 Diabetes: A prospective, randomized, placebo-controlled study. *Diabetes Care*, janvier. https://doi.org/10.2337/dc12-1371.

Davis, A., M. Christiansen, J. F. Horowitz, S. Klein, M. K. Hellerstein, and R. E. Ostlund. 2000. Effect of Pinitol Treatment on Insulin Action in Subjects with Insulin Resistance. *Diabetes Care* 23 (7): 1000-1005.

D'Oria, R., L. Laviola, F. Giorgino, V. Unfer, S. Bettocchi, and M. Scioscia. 2017. PKB/Akt and MAPK/ERK Phosphorylation Is Highly Induced by Inositols: Novel Potential Insights in Endothelial Dysfunction in Preeclampsia. *Pregnancy Hypertension* 10 (Octobre): 107‑12. https://doi.org/10.1016/j.preghy.2017.07.001.

Esposito, K., M. Ciotola, D. Carleo, B. Schisano, F. Saccomanno, F. C. Sasso, D. Cozzolino, R. Assaloni, D. Merante, A. Ceriello, and D. Giugliano. 2006a. Effect of rosiglitazone on endothelial function and inflammatory markers in patients with the metabolic syndrome. *Diabetes Care* 29 (5): 1071‑76. https://doi.org/10.2337/diacare.2951071.

Farias, V. X., F. H. P. Macêdo, M. B. Oquendo, A. R. Tomé, S. N. Báo, D. O. S. Cintra, C. F. Santos, A. A. Albuquerque, D. B. Heimark, J. Larner, M. C. Fonteles, J. H. Leal-Cardoso, and N. R. Nascimento. 2011. Chronic Treatment with D-Chiro-Inositol Prevents Autonomic and Somatic Neuropathy in STZ-Induced Diabetic Mice. *Diabetes, Obesity & Metabolism* 13 (3): 243‑50. https://doi.org/10.1111/j.1463-1326.2010.01344.x.

Farren, M., N. Daly, A. McKeating, B. Kinsley, M. J. Turner, and S. Daly. 2017. The Prevention of Gestational Diabetes Mellitus with Antenatal Oral Inositol Supplementation: A Randomized Controlled Trial. *Diabetes Care* 40 (6): 759‑63. https://doi.org/10.2337/dc16-2449.

Fontbonne, A., I. Diouf, M. Baccara-Dinet, E. Eschwege, andM.-A. Charles. 2009. Effects of 1-Year Treatment with Metformin on Metabolic and Cardiovascular Risk Factors in Non-Diabetic Upper-Body Obese Subjects with Mild Glucose Anomalies: A Post-Hoc Analysis of the BIGPRO1 Trial. *Diabetes & Metabolism* 35 (5): 385‑91. https://doi.org/10.1016/j.diabet.2009.03.005.

Fonteles, M. C., M. Q. Almeida, and J. Larner. 2000. Antihyperglycemic Effects of 3-O-Methyl-D-Chiro-Inositol and D-Chiro-Inositol Associated with Manganese in Streptozotocin Diabetic Rats. *Hormone and Metabolic Research* [*Hormon- Und Stoffwechselforschung*] 32 (4): 129‑32. https://doi.org/10.1055/s-2007-978606.

Fonteles, M. C., L. C. Huang, and J. Larner. 1996. Infusion of PH 2.0 D-Chiro-Inositol Glycan Insulin Putative Mediator Normalizes Plasma Glucose in Streptozotocin Diabetic Rats at a Dose Equivalent to Insulin without Inducing Hypoglycaemia. *Diabetologia* 39 (6): 731‑34.

Frick, W., A. Bauer, J. Bauer, S. Wied, and G. Müller. 1998a. Structure-Activity Relationship of Synthetic Phosphoinositolglycans Mimicking Metabolic Insulin Action. *Biochemistry* 37 (38): 13421-36. https://doi.org/10.1021/bi9806201.

Frick, W., A. Bauer, J. Bauer, S. Wied, and G. Müller. 1998b. Insulin-Mimetic Signalling of Synthetic Phosphoinositolglycans in Isolated Rat Adipocytes. *The Biochemical Journal* 336 (Pt 1) (novembre): 163-81.

Gao, Y. F., M. N. Zhang, T. X. Wang, T. C. Wu, R. D. Ai, and Z. S. Zhang. 2016. Hypoglycemic Effect of D-Chiro-Inositol in Type 2 Diabetes Mellitus Rats through the PI3K/Akt Signaling Pathway. *Molecular and Cellular Endocrinology* 433: 26-34. https://doi.org/10.1016/j.mce.2016.05.013.

Geethan, P. K. M. Anu, and P. S. M. Prince. 2008. Antihyperlipidemic Effect of D-Pinitol on Streptozotocin-Induced Diabetic Wistar Rats. *Journal of Biochemical and Molecular Toxicology* 22 (4): 220-24. https://doi.org/10.1002/jbt.20218.

Giordano, D., F. Corrado, A. Santamaria, S. Quattrone, B. Pintaudi, A. Di Benedetto, and R. D'Anna. 2011. Effects of Myo-Inositol Supplementation in Postmenopausal Women with Metabolic Syndrome: A Perspective, Randomized, Placebo-Controlled Study. *Menopause* (New York, N.Y.) 18 (1): 102-4. https://doi.org/10.1097/gme.0b013e3181e8e1b1.

Greene, D. A., P. V. De Jesus, and A. I. Winegrad. 1975. Effects of Insulin and Dietary Myoinositol on Impaired Peripheral Motor Nerve Conduction Velocity in Acute Streptozotocin Diabetes. *The Journal of Clinical Investigation* 55 (6): 1326-36. https://doi.org/10.1172/JCI108052.

Gupta, A. K., S. R. Smith, F. L. Greenway, and G. A. Bray. 2009. Pioglitazone Treatment in Type 2 Diabetes Mellitus When Combined with Portion Control Diet Modifies the Metabolic Syndrome. *Diabetes, Obesity & Metabolism* 11 (4): 330-37. https://doi.org/10.1111/j.1463-1326.2008.00965.x.

Hecht, M. L., Y. H. Tsai, X. Liu, C. Wolfrum, and P. H. Seeberger. 2010. Synthetic Inositol Phosphoglycans Related to GPI Lack Insulin-Mimetic Activity. *ACS Chemical Biology* 5 (11): 1075-86. https://doi.org/10.1021/cb1002152.

Hong, J. H., H. W. Jang, Y. E. Kang, J. H. Lee, K. S. Kim, H. J. Kim, K. R. Park, and B. J. Ku. 2012. Urinary Chiro- and Myo-Inositol Levels as a Biological Marker for Type 2 Diabetes Mellitus. *Disease Markers* 33 (4): 193-99. https://doi.org/10.3233/DMA-2012-0925.

Kang, M. J., J. I. Kim, S. Y. Yoon, J. C. Kim, and I. J. Cha. 2006. Pinitol from Soybeans Reduces Postprandial Blood Glucose in Patients with Type 2 Diabetes Mellitus. *Journal of Medicinal Food* 9 (2): 182-86. https://doi.org/10.1089/jmf.2006.9.182.

Khandelwal, M., E. A. Reece, Y. K. Wu, and M. Borenstein. 1998. Dietary Myo-Inositol Therapy in Hyperglycemia-Induced Embryopathy. *Teratology* 57 (2): 79-84. https://doi.org/10.1002/(SICI)1096-9926(199802)57:2<79::AID-TERA6>3.0.CO;2-1.

Kim, H. J., K. S. Park, S. K. Lee, K. W. Min, K. A. Han, Y. K. Kim, and B. J. Ku. 2012. Effects of Pinitol on Glycemic Control, Insulin Resistance and Adipocytokine Levels in Patients with Type 2 Diabetes Mellitus. *Annals of Nutrition & Metabolism* 60 (1): 1-5. https://doi.org/10.1159/000334834.

Kim, J. I., J. C. Kim, M. J. Kang, M. S. Lee, J. J. Kim, and I. J. Cha. 2005. Effects of Pinitol Isolated from Soybeans on Glycaemic Control and Cardiovascular Risk Factors in Korean Patients with Type II Diabetes Mellitus: A Randomized Controlled Study. *European Journal of Clinical Nutrition* 59 (3): 456-58. https://doi.org/10.1038/sj.ejcn.1602081.

Larner, J. 2001. D-Chiro-Inositol in Insulin Action and Insulin Resistance-Old-Fashioned Biochemistry Still at Work. *IUBMB Life* 51 (3): 139-48. https://doi.org/10.1080/152165401753544205.

Larner, J. 2002. D-Chiro-Inositol--Its Functional Role in Insulin Action and Its Deficit in Insulin Resistance. *International Journal of Experimental Diabetes Research* 3 (1): 47-60.

Larner, J., D. L. Brautigan, and M. O. Thorner. 2010. D-Chiro-Inositol Glycans in Insulin Signaling and Insulin Resistance. *Molecular Medicine* (Cambridge, Mass.) 16 (11‑12): 543‑52. https://doi.org/10.2119/molmed.2010.00107.

Lazarenko, R., J. Geisler, D. Bayliss, J. Larner, and C. Li. 2014. D-Chiro-Inositol Glycan Stimulates Insulin Secretion in Pancreatic β Cells. *Molecular and Cellular Endocrinology* 387 (1‑2): 1‑7. https://doi.org/10.1016/j.mce.2014.02.004.

Li, X. W., Y. Liu, W. Hao, and J. R Yang. 2014. Sequoyitol Ameliorates Diabetic Nephropathy in Diabetic Rats Induced with a High-Fat Diet and a Low Dose of Streptozotocin. *Canadian Journal of Physiology and Pharmacology* 92 (5): 405‑17. https://doi.org/10.1139/cjpp-2013-0307.

Lubin, V., R. Shojai, P. Darmon, and E. Cosson. 2016. A Pilot Study of Gestational Diabetes Mellitus Not Controlled by Diet Alone: First-Line Medical Treatment with Myoinositol May Limit the Need for Insulin. *Diabetes & Metabolism* 42 (3): 192‑95. https://doi.org/10.1016/j.diabet.2016.01.005.

Maeba, R., H. Hara, H. Ishikawa, S. Hayashi, N. Yoshimura, J. Kusano, Y. Takeoka, D. Yasuda, T. Okazaki, M. Kinoshita, and T. Teramoto. 2008. Myo-Inositol Treatment Increases Serum Plasmalogens and Decreases Small Dense LDL, Particularly in Hyperlipidemic Subjects with Metabolic Syndrome. *Journal of Nutritional Science and Vitaminology* 54 (3): 196‑202.

Matarrelli, B., E. Vitacolonna, M. D'Angelo, G. Pavone, P. A. Mattei, M. Liberati, and C. Celentano. 2013. Effect of Dietary Myo-Inositol Supplementation in Pregnancy on the Incidence of Maternal Gestational Diabetes Mellitus and Fetal Outcomes: A Randomized Controlled Trial. *The Journal of Maternal-Fetal & Neonatal Medicine: The Official Journal of the European Association of Perinatal Medicine, the Federation of Asia and Oceania Perinatal Societies, the International Society of Perinatal Obstetricians* 26 (10): 967‑72. https://doi.org/10.3109/14767058.2013.766691.

Maurizi, A. R., M. Menduni, R. Del Toro, S. Kyanvash, D. Maggi, C. Guglielmi, A. L. Pantano, G. Defeudis, E. Fioriti, S. Manfrini, and P. Pozzilli. 2017. A Pilot Study of D-Chiro-Inositol plus Folic Acid in Overweight Patients with Type 1 Diabetes. *Acta Diabetologica* 54 (4): 361‑65. https://doi.org/10.1007/s00592-016-0954-x.

Muscogiuri, G., S. Palomba, A. S. Laganà, and F. Orio. 2016. Inositols in the Treatment of Insulin-Mediated Diseases. *International Journal of Endocrinology* 2016: 3058393. https://doi.org/10.1155/2016/3058393.

Ortmeyer, H. K., N. L. Bodkin, K. Lilley, J. Larner, and B. C. Hansen. 1993. Chiroinositol Deficiency and Insulin Resistance. I. Urinary Excretion Rate of Chiroinositol Is Directly Associated with Insulin Resistance in Spontaneously Diabetic Rhesus Monkeys. *Endocrinology* 132 (2): 640‑45. https://doi.org/10.1210/endo.132.2.8425483.

Ortmeyer, H. K., L. C. Huang, L. Zhang, B. C. Hansen, and J. Larner. 1993. Chiroinositol Deficiency and Insulin Resistance. II. Acute Effects of D-Chiroinositol Administration in Streptozotocin-Diabetic Rats, Normal Rats given a Glucose Load, and Spontaneously Insulin-Resistant Rhesus Monkeys. *Endocrinology* 132 (2): 646‑51. https://doi.org/10.1210/endo.132.2.8425484.

Paul, C., A. S. Laganà, P. Maniglio, O. Triolo, and D. M. Brady. 2016. Inositol's and Other Nutraceuticals' Synergistic Actions Counteract Insulin Resistance in Polycystic Ovarian Syndrome and Metabolic Syndrome: State-of-the-Art and Future Perspectives. *Gynecological Endocrinology: The Official Journal of the International Society of Gynecological Endocrinology* 32 (6): 431‑38. https://doi.org/10.3109/09513590.2016.1144741.

Petersen, K. F., and G. I. Shulman. 2006. Etiology of Insulin Resistance. *The American Journal of Medicine* 119 (5 Suppl 1): S10-16. https://doi.org/10.1016/j.amjmed.2006.01.009.

Pintaudi, B., and G. Di Vieste. 2017. Comment on Farren et al. The Prevention of Gestational Diabetes Mellitus with Antenatal Oral Inositol Supplementation: A Randomized Controlled Trial. Diabetes Care 2017;40:759–763. *Diabetes Care* 40 (12):e172.

Plourde, R., M. D'Alarcao, and A. R. Saltiel. 1992. Synthesis and characterization of an insulin-mimetic disaccharide. *The Journal of Organic Chemistry* 57 (9): 2606‑10. https://doi.org/10.1021/jo00035a015.

Plows, J. F., F. Budin, R. A. M. Andersson, V. J. Mills, K. Mace, S. T. Davidge, M. H. Vickers, P. N. Baker, I. Silva-Zolezzi, and J. L. Stanley. 2017. The Effects of Myo-Inositol and B and D Vitamin Supplementation in the Db/+ Mouse Model of Gestational Diabetes Mellitus. *Nutrients* 9 (2). https://doi.org/10.3390/nu9020141.

Reaven, G. M. 2006. The Metabolic Syndrome: Is This Diagnosis Necessary? *The American Journal of Clinical Nutrition* 83 (6): 1237‑47. https://doi.org/10.1093/ajcn/83.6.1237.

Reddy, K. K., J. R. Falck, and J. Capdevila. 1993. Insulin second messengers: Synthesis of 6-O-(2-amino-2-deoxy-α-D-glucopyranosyl)-D-chiro-inositol-1-phosphate. *Tetrahedron Letters*, The International Journal for the Rapid Publication of Preliminary, 34 (49): 7869‑72. https://doi.org/10.1016/S0040-4039(00)61497-1.

Reece, E. A., M. Khandelwal, Y. K. Wu, and M. Borenstein. 1997. Dietary Intake of Myo-Inositol and Neural Tube Defects in Offspring of Diabetic Rats. *American Journal of Obstetrics and Gynecology* 176 (3): 536‑39.

Samuel, V. T., and G. I. Shulman. 2012. Mechanisms for Insulin Resistance: Common Threads and Missing Links. *Cell* 148 (5): 852‑71. https://doi.org/10.1016/j.cell.2012.02.017.

Santamaria, A., D. Giordano, F. Corrado, B. Pintaudi, M. L. Interdonato, G. Di Vieste, A. Di Benedetto, and R. D'Anna. 2012. One-Year Effects of Myo-Inositol Supplementation in Postmenopausal Women with Metabolic Syndrome. *Climacteric: The Journal of the International Menopause Society* 15 (5): 490‑95. https://doi.org/10.3109/13697137.2011.631063.

Santamaria, A., A. Di Benedetto, E. Petrella, B. Pintaudi, F. Corrado, R. D'Anna, I. Neri, and F. Facchinetti. 2016. Myo-Inositol May Prevent Gestational Diabetes Onset in Overweight Women: A Randomized,

Controlled Trial. *The Journal of Maternal-Fetal & Neonatal Medicine: The Official Journal of the European Association of Perinatal Medicine, the Federation of Asia and Oceania Perinatal Societies, the International Society of Perinatal Obstetricians* 29 (19): 3234‑37. https://doi.org/10.3109/14767058.2015.1121478.

Shen, H., M. Shao, K. W. Cho, S. Wang, Z. Chen, L. Sheng, T. Wang, Y. Liu, and L. Rui. 2012. Herbal Constituent Sequoyitol Improves Hyperglycemia and Glucose Intolerance by Targeting Hepatocytes, Adipocytes, and β-Cells. *American Journal of Physiology. Endocrinology and Metabolism* 302 (8): E932-940. https://doi.org/10.1152/ajpendo.00479.2011.

Sivakumar, S., P. Palsamy, and S. P. Subramanian. 2010a. Attenuation of Oxidative Stress and Alteration of Hepatic Tissue Ultrastructure by D-Pinitol in Streptozotocin-Induced Diabetic Rats. *Free Radical Research* 44 (6): 668‑78. https://doi.org/10.3109/10715761003733901.

Sivakumar, S., P. Palsamy, and S. P. Subramanian. 2010b. Impact of D-Pinitol on the Attenuation of Proinflammatory Cytokines, Hyperglycemia-Mediated Oxidative Stress and Protection of Kidney Tissue Ultrastructure in Streptozotocin-Induced Diabetic Rats. *Chemico-Biological Interactions* 188 (1): 237‑45. https://doi.org/10.1016/j.cbi.2010.07.014.

Sivakumar, S., and S. P.Subramanian. 2009. Pancreatic Tissue Protective Nature of D-Pinitol Studied in Streptozotocin-Mediated Oxidative Stress in Experimental Diabetic Rats. *European Journal of Pharmacology* 622 (1‑3): 65‑70. https://doi.org/10.1016/j.ejphar.2009.09.021.

Suzuki, S., C. Suzuki, Y. Hinokio, Y. Ishigaki, H. Katagiri, M. Kanzaki, V. N. Azev, N. Chakraborty, and M. d'Alarcao. 2014. Insulin-Mimicking Bioactivities of Acylated Inositol Glycans in Several Mouse Models of Diabetes with or without Obesity. *PloS One* 9 (6): e100466. https://doi.org/10.1371/journal.pone.0100466.

Yamakoshi, M., and S. Kawazu. 2008. Lucica MI Urinary Myoinositol Kit: A New Diagnostic Test for Diabetes Mellitus and Glucose Intolerance. *Molecular Diagnosis & Therapy* 12 (3): 189-91.

Yao, Y., F. Shan, J. Bian, F. Chen, M. Wang, and G. Ren. 2008. D-Chiro-Inositol-Enriched Tartary Buckwheat Bran Extract Lowers the Blood Glucose Level in KK-Ay Mice. *Journal of Agricultural and Food Chemistry* 56 (21): 10027-31. https://doi.org/10.1021/jf801879m.

Zheng, X., Z. Liu, Y. Zhang, Y. Lin, J. Song, L. Zheng, and S. Lin. 2015. Relationship Between Myo-Inositol Supplementary and Gestational Diabetes Mellitus: A Meta-Analysis. *Medicine* 94 (42): e1604. https://doi.org/10.1097/MD.0000000000001604.

In: Inositols
Editor: Vittorio Unfer
ISBN: 978-1-53614-912-8

Chapter 5

INOSITOLS AND GESTATIONAL DIABETES

Angelo Santamaria, MD and Rosario D'Anna*, MD

Department of Human Pathology,
University of Messina, Messina ME, Italy

ABSTRACT

Gestational diabetes mellitus (GDM) is defined as a carbohydrate intolerance first recognized during pregnancy. It is associated with increased risks such as caesarean delivery, hypertensive disorders, and development of type 2 diabetes later in life for the mother, as well as macrosomia, shoulder dystocia, hypoglycemia, respiratory distress syndrome, and obesity for the newborn. Recently the involvement of myo-inositol in the mechanisms of glycemic control preventing GDM occurrence in women with a family history of type 2 diabetes has been shown. It has been reported also that myo-inositol may reduce insulin resistance in women affected by GDM. Therefore, the interest of clinicians and researchers is widely increasing and it will be discussed throughout this chapter.

* Corresponding Author's Email: rdanna@unime.it.

Keywords: inositol, myo-inositol, d-chiro-inositol, gestational diabetes, insulin resistance

INTRODUCTION

Pregnancy is a condition of physiological insulin resistance that presumably allows the fetus to receive more nutrients from the mother, especially in the third trimester of pregnancy. Maternal postprandial hyperglycemia provides the fetus with carbohydrates and amino acids through the placenta by facilitated carrier transport (Buchanan et al. 1990). When the mother is unable to compensate glucose post-prandial load with an increased pancreatic insulin secretion, Gestational Diabetes Mellitus (GDM) develops (Catalano et al. 1999). The molecular mechanism underlying insulin resistance in GDM is still poorly understood, although some authors explain this condition as an impairment of a second messenger of the intracellular insulin pathway (Buchanan and Xiang 2005). Insulin resistance is not a single-gene disorder; researchers have identified numerous genes with alleles that can make people more likely to develop insulin resistance (Pedersen 1999, Virkamäki, Ueki, and Kahn 1999). Unfavorable diet and sedentary lifestyle may also contribute. Insulin resistance appears to be determined by a polygenic model of susceptibility where particular mutations do not totally impair gene function but result in mild compromise, which becomes overt when several gene mutations or external conditions are combined. Fetal hyperinsulinemia, as a direct consequence of maternal fetal hyperglycemia, explains the main clinical features of GDM, such as fetal macrosomia and supports the central role of insulin resistance in the pathogenesis of the syndrome. For this reason, GDM is defined as "carbohydrate intolerance of varying degree of severity with onset or first recognition during pregnancy" (Metzger and Coustan, 1998). It is the most common medical complication and metabolic disorder of pregnancy (Carr and Gabbe 1998).

According to the clinical guidelines for the management of diabetes in pregnancy, the screening and diagnosis of GDM should be undertaken between the 24th and 28th week of pregnancy, but vary from country to country (NICE, 2015). Furthermore, in some countries screening is based on different risk factors. Development of GDM depends on a number of risk factors such as: 1) previous GDM; 2) previously elevated blood glucose level; 3) ethnicity; 4) age ≥ 40 years; 5) family history of diabetes mellitus or diabetes; 6) obesity, 7) previous macrosomia; 8) polycystic ovarian syndrome; 9) pregnancy weight gain. GDM is the most common medical problem of pregnancy and is related to an increased risk of complications in pregnancy, including fetal macrosomia, birth trauma, neonatal hypoglycemia and hyperbilirubinemia, cesarean section, and hypertensive syndromes (Langer et al. 2005). Furthermore, for these women there is an increased risk of glucose intolerance later in life, and 35-60% of women affected by GDM develop type 2 diabetes within 10 years from the index pregnancy (Metzger et al. 2007). Moreover, the offspring of GDM mothers have an increased prevalence of obesity, type 2 diabetes, and cardiovascular disease in their adult life (Dabelea 2007, Lee et al. 2007). The wide range of GDM prevalence depends on the prevalence of insulin resistance and type 2 diabetes in the population considered, but also on the different diagnostic tests employed. Recently, the International Association of Diabetes in Pregnancy Study Groups (IADPSG) proposed new criteria with the aim to resolve the lack of uniform criteria for GDM diagnosis (International Association of Diabetes and Pregnancy Study Groups, Consensus 2010). These suggestions derive from the published results of the Hyperglycemia and Adverse Pregnancy Outcome (HAPO) Study, a multicenter double blind observational study in which glucose value of the Oral Glucose Tolerance Test (OGTT) were correlated with the obstetrical outcomes (Group 2008). Subsequently, the IADPSG panel proposed a universal 75 g-OGTT at 24-28 weeks of gestation, with new thresholds calculated at a predefined level of glucose associated with a 1.75 odds ratio (OR) increased risk (compared to median glucose values) for each of the outcomes considered (birth weight >90th percentile, cord C-peptide >90th percentile, and percent of body fat >90th percentile). These new calculated thresholds are 92 mg/dL (fasting), 180 mg/dL (after 1 h), and 153 mg/dL (after 2 h). If one of these values is equal or exceed the established threshold, GDM is diagnosed. Accepting the new criteria, the number of pregnant women affected became almost double with an increase of healthcare cost. There is also concern about medicalization of potentially healthy pregnant women. For these reasons, in several countries the healthcare systems are still reluctant to adopt these new criteria. Hence, GDM is a rising problem worldwide and the identification of effective therapeutic approaches for preventing GDM is of great importance. Both nonpharmacological and pharmacological ways to counteract GDM are taken in consideration by clinicians.

Current Management of GDM

Interventions like diet and exercise are the mainstay of treatment in GDM (American Diabetes Association 2015, Shepherd et al. 2017). When diet and lifestyle changes fail to control the euglycemic state, pharmaceutical interventions are undertaken. Traditionally, insulin, metformin, and glyburide are the predominant approaches for the management of blood glucose in pregnant women; most oral agents cross the placenta or lack long-term safety data (American Diabetes Association 2015).

Insulin therapy is widely used during pregnancy in women with type 1 diabetes for optimal glycemic control, but also with type 2 diabetes. Less commonly, is given to pregnant women with GDM, however, balancing the insulin while eating is useful to keep the glucose levels in the normal range. Even though insulin has been considered safe during pregnancy, there is not enough evidence yet, or are poorly reported, for the long-term maternal and neonatal outcomes (Brown et al. 2017). Moreover, few studies reported that exogenous insulin might slightly affect placental, fetal and maternal outcomes in patients with GDM (Arshad, Karim, and Ara Hasan 2014, Brown et al. 2017).

Metformin, a biguanide anti-diabetic oral drug, currently is the first-line therapy for type 2 diabetes in many countries (Nankervis and Conn 2013). It is recommended as monotherapy by the American Diabetes Association clinical practice guidelines, for the initial glucose-lowering activity, considering the addition to other adjuvant treatments depending on efficacy, risk of hypoglycaemia, weight, side-effects, and costs (American Diabetes Association 2016). It reduces blood glucose concentration by mechanisms different from those of insulin secretagogues or exogenous insulin therapy; it reduces hepatic glucose output and increases insulin sensitivity.

Clinical experience has shown the beneficial use of metformin in treating GDM, however its administration during pregnancy is controversial (Feig and Moses 2011, Gray et al. 2017). Considerable research using metformin has been done on pregnant women with polycystic ovary syndrome (PCOS), with contrasting results (Glueck et al. 2008, Tang et al. 2012, Ainuddin et al. 2015, Glueck et al. 2003). Recently, in obese pregnant women was observed that fasting glucose and insulin were lower at 28 weeks' gestation in the group using metformin, but no difference in the risk of developing gestational diabetes was reported, by either IADSPG or WHO (World Health Organization) criteria, between supplementation of metformin or placebo (Chiswick et al. 2015). Despite short term maternal and neonatal safety measures, the absence of long-term safety data in offspring and the gastrointestinal-directed action of metformin might discourage pregnant women to undertake this treatment.

After a peculiar research in the literature, it can be said that diverse and suitable options for the management of GDM have been tested so far; however, further trials in the prevention and/or treatment of GDM are encouraged.

Inositols in Clinical Practice

A growing body of research is currently focused on the role of inositol isomers, and in particular myo-inositol (MI) and D-chiroinositol (DCI). In vivo conversion of MI to the other isomer DCI can occur in tissues expressing the specific epimerase. Both have been shown to exert insulin-mimetic action and to lower postprandial glucose, principally as components of glycosyl-phosphatidylinositol (GPI) and of inositol phosphoglycans (IPGs) that would constitute second messengers of insulin action in the GPI/IPG pathway. Furthermore, it has been shown that MI-PG and DCI-PG mediate different actions of insulin: MI-PG is involved in cellular glucose uptake via activation of Glucose Transporter Type 4 (GLUT-4) translocation to the plasma membranes and so enhancing glucose entry into the cells; whereas DCI-PG is involved in glycogen synthesis. It has been shown that in human subjects diabetes mellitus (DM) is characterized by an imbalance between MI and DCI, with an increased urinary excretion of MI (Kennington et al. 1990). These results suggest that in DM a MI intracellular depletion occurs, probably caused by an inhibition of cellular MI uptake because of a competition between MI and glucose since MI and glucose have structural similarities (Haneda et al. 1990). Therefore, high glucose concentration in the extracellular space could impair MI uptake and so contribute to the MI intra-cellular depletion observed in DM. Depletion of intracellular MI and consequently decreased production of DCI from MI reduces the availability of these 2 substances for their incorporation into IPGs, putative second messengers of insulin. Therefore, the decreased inositol content in insulin target tissues could reduce insulin signal transduction involving IPGs and so further enhance or contribute to the insulin resistance in those tissues. First studies with inositols have been carried out successfully in women affected by PCOS, a condition characterized by insulin resistance too (Baillargeon et al. 2006, Gerli et al. 2007). These observations suggested that insulin resistance in GDM, as in PCOS, might be improved by inositol administration. Thus, MI supplementation was used in the treatment of women with a diagnosis of GDM (Corrado et al. 2011). During the study period, 84 consecutive women with GDM were randomly assigned to receive diet and 400 mcg of folic acid alone or diet, folic acid, and MI (2 g/twice a day). Blood samples were collected to determine the markers of insulin resistance (HOMA-IR and adiponectin) at the time of the OGTT, and then repeated after 8 weeks of treatment. The markers improved in both groups, but the delta decrease was greater in the inositol-treated group, and the differences between the two groups were significant (HOMA-IR $p=0.0001$; adiponectin $p=0.009$). Recently, another experience (Fraticelli et al. 2018) has been carried out on women with GDM randomized and assigned to one of the four arms of the study (n.20 per arm) to receive daily: 400 mcg folic acid (control treatment),

4000 mg MI plus 400 mcg folic acid (MI treatment), 500 mg DCI plus 400 mcg folic acid (DCI treatment) or 1100/27.6 mg MI/DCI plus 400 mcg folic acid (MI plus DCI treatment). The homeostasis model assessment of insulin resistance (HOMA-IR) was measured at the diagnosis of GDM and after 8 weeks of treatment. Secondary outcomes, obstetric outcomes and any maternal or fetal complications at delivery were also collected. A significant delta decrease in HOMA-IR index was found in subjects of MI group without insulin therapy compared to the control group ($p < 0.001$). A lower variation in average weight gain (at delivery vs pre-pregnancy and OGTT period) was detected in MI group vs control group ($p = 0.001$ and $p = 0.019$, respectively). Moreover, women exposed to MI and MI plus DCI required a significantly lower necessity of an intensified insulin treatment. Women of the control group had newborns with higher birth weight compared with women treated with inositol ($p = 0.032$). A possible use of MI in preventing GDM came from a retrospective study which involved a group of 98 women with PCOS who had a pregnancy during the assumption of MI or metformin (D'anna et al. 2012). The women treated with a MI regimen (4 g/day plus folic acid 400 mcg/day) were supplemented until delivery, while women treated with metformin regimen stopped the drug as soon as pregnancy was diagnosed and were considered controls. The OGTT was performed at 24-28 weeks of pregnancy according to the Carpenter and Coustan criteria (Carpenter and Coustan 1982). The prevalence of GDM was 17% in the MI group compared to 54% in the controls, with an OR of 2.4 (CI 95%, 1.3-4.4). This little study suggested that MI could be used also to prevent GDM; thus 3 prospective, randomized, placebo-controlled studies were carried out enrolling women with different risk factors: a) a parent with type 2 diabetes (D'Anna et al. 2013); b) obese: body mass index (BMI) ≥ 30 kg/m2 (D'Anna et al. 2015); c) overweight: BMI from 25.0 to 29.9 kg/m^2 (Santamaria et al. 2016). In all these studies the same dosage was used: MI (2 g plus 200 mcg folic acid twice a day) or placebo (200 mcg folic acid twice a day) from the end of the first trimester until delivery, and the same number of women enrolled (110 in each arm). Despite the different risk factor considered in the inclusion criteria, the reduction of GDM rate in each study was similar, statistically significant and more than 60%. Whether the result of the primary outcome (decreased GDM rate in the group treated with MI) was encouraging, secondary outcomes related to the reduction of GDM complications (macrosomia, gestational hypertension and pre-term birth) were not satisfactory, probably for their low prevalence. Thus, a secondary analysis on the 3 databases related to the 3 RCT's trials was performed involving a total of 660 women (Santamaria et al. 2018). This very recent study has shown that MI is not only effective in GDM reduction rate (Figure 1), but it's also effective in decreasing the incidence of pre-term birth, macrosomia and Large for Gestational Age (LGA) fetuses significantly (Figure 2) (Santamaria et al. 2018).

Other studies have subsequently been carried out to explore the possibility that MI might prevent GDM. Another group (Matarrelli et al. 2013) performed a small prospective, randomized controlled study on women with another important risk factor: elevated first-trimester fasting glucose (> 100 mg/dl), reporting a reduced risk of developing GDM in the group treated with MI (OR 0.12) at the same dosage of previous studies. The efficacy of MI seems to be dose-effective because in another RCT study, in the group supplemented daily with a combination of 1,100 mg MI and 27,6 mg of DCI and 400 mcg of folic acid, there was no difference in GDM rate compared to the placebo group (Farren et al. 2017). However, the effective dosage of MI usually used is safe and well tolerated. Side effects, when present, are mild and mainly gastrointestinal like nausea, flatus and diarrhea (Carlomagno and Unfer 2011). Furthermore, it is clearly assessed that MI transfer from the mother to the fetus is very low with no potential damage for the fetus (Coustan 2013).

A recent Cochrane review evaluated in total four randomised controlled trials, assessing the effects of MI for the prevention of GDM (Crawford et al. 2015). Dietary supplementation with MI during pregnancy was associated with a reduction in the incidence of GDM compared with control (risk ratio (RR) 0.43, 95% confidence interval (CI) 0.29 to 0.64; three trials; n = 502 women). However, all these studies included were carried out in Italy, therefore novel trials involving pregnant women of different ethnicities are encouraged.

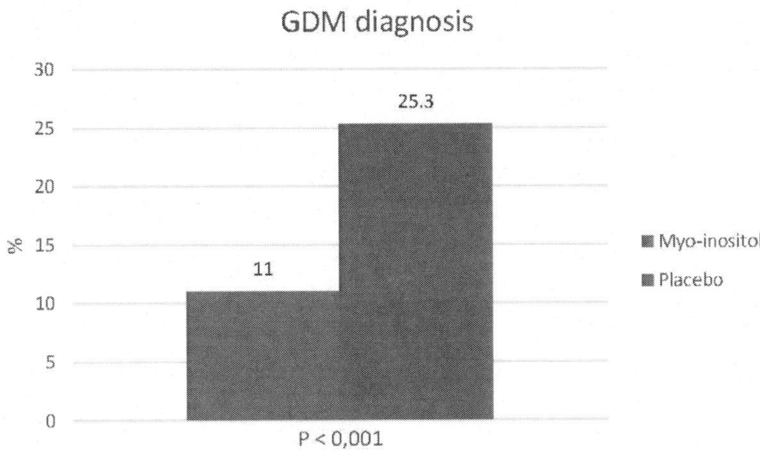

Figure 1. Incidence of GDM in both groups.

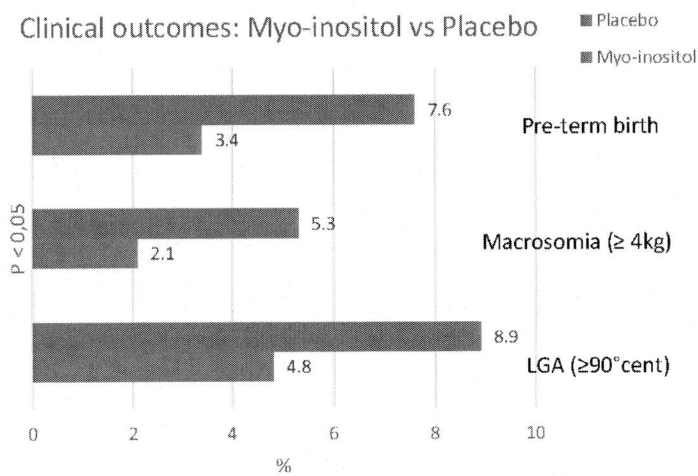

Figure 2. Clinical outcomes in both groups.

Furthermore, a systematic review and meta-analysis evaluated the effect of MI in preventing GDM (Zhang et al. 2018). The meta-analysis of five randomized controlled trials reported that MI supplementation significantly reduced the incidence of GDM (risk ratio (RR) = 0.43; 95%CI = 0.21–0.89; p = 0.02). Another meta-analysis confirmed the effectiveness of MI, compared with placebo, in lowering the incidence of GDM, in pregnant women with high risk (RR = 0.44, 95% CI [0.32, 0.62], $P < 0.0001$) (Guo et al. 2017). Here, the pooled results expressed as mean difference (MD) reported that the supplementation of MI significantly lowers fasting OGTT (MD = -0.18, 95% CI [-0.24, -0.12], $P < 0.00001$), 1h OGTT (MD = -0.55, 95% CI [-0.81, -0.28], $P < 0.00001$), and 2h OGTT (MD = -0.58, 95% CI [-0.94, -0.23], $P = 0.001$) at approximately 26 weeks of gestational age. However further analysis on secondary outcomes such as lower birth weight after MI supplementation is required.

Interestingly, a case report showed great results on the supplementation of MI in a 29-year-old Caucasian woman, nulliparous, affected by GDM (Costabile and Unfer 2017). After treatment with 4 g of MI 3 times per day for 3 weeks, combined with a low-calorie diet, the patient showed a significant decrease of glycemia in a faster and steady way at fasting, 1-hour and 2-hours after-meal. The safety profile of MI at this high dosage, free from any side effects, confirmed its safety during pregnancy. Furthermore, MI reduced the blood glucose levels in a short-time of administration. This result, even only preliminary and in one only case may open future prospectives for a safe and effective therapy for GDM.

Analyzing all these findings, it can be summarized that among inositols, the clinical experience with MI in reducing GDM rate seems until now the only effective.

CONCLUSION

In conclusion, MI intake from the early stages of pregnancy in overweight women has been shown to decrease the incidence of GDM. This statement is confirmed by two recent meta-analysis (Guo et al. 2017, Zhang et al. 2018). In the literature, different studies can be found outlining the role of MI in reducing GDM rate in women at risk. However, large, well-designed, randomized, double blind studies are needed to confirm the beneficial effect of this supplement. Even though the safety of this molecule has now been widely accepted (Carlomagno and Unfer 2011) further clinical evidences and analysis during pregnancy assessing adverse effects and the maternal and fetal long-term effects of this intervention should be considered. It would be also interesting, to assess clinical trial to evaluate the effectiveness of MI not only in preventing but also in treating GDM. This might open a new scenario for the management of this condition.

Conflict of Interest

None.

References

Ainuddin, J. A., S. Kazi, S. Aftab, and A. Kamran. 2015. "Metformin for preventing gestational diabetes in women with polycystic ovarian syndrome." *J Coll Physicians Surg Pak* 25 (4):237-41. doi: 04.2015/jcpsp.237241.

American Diabetes Association. 2015. "12. Management of Diabetes in Pregnancy." *Diabetes Care* 38 (Supplement 1):S77.

American Diabetes Association. 2016. "7. Approaches to glycemic treatment." *Diabetes Care* 39 (Supplement 1):S52-S59.

Arshad, R., N. Karim, and J. A. Hasan. 2014. "Effects of insulin on placental, fetal and maternal outcomes in gestational diabetes mellitus." *Pakistan Journal of Medical Sciences* 30 (2):240-244.

Baillargeon, J. P., E. Diamanti-Kandarakis, R. E. Ostlund, Jr., T. Apridonidze, M. J. Iuorno, and J. E. Nestler. 2006. "Altered D-chiro-inositol urinary clearance in women with polycystic ovary syndrome." *Diabetes Care* 29 (2):300-5.

Brown, J., L. Grzeskowiak, K. Williamson, M. R. Downie, and C. A. Crowther. 2017. "Insulin for the treatment of women with gestational diabetes." *Cochrane Database Syst Rev* 11:Cd012037. doi: 10.1002/14651858.CD012037.pub2.

Buchanan, T. A., B. E. Metzger, N. Freinkel, and R. N. Bergman. 1990. "Insulin sensitivity and B-cell responsiveness to glucose during late pregnancy in lean and moderately obese women with normal glucose tolerance or mild gestational diabetes." *American Journal of Obstetrics & Gynecology* 162 (4):1008-1014.

Buchanan, T. A., and Anny H. Xiang. 2005. "Gestational diabetes mellitus." *The Journal of Clinical Investigation* 115 (3):485-491.

Carlomagno, G., and V. Unfer. 2011. "Inositol safety: clinical evidences." *Eur Rev Med Pharmacol Sci* 15 (8):931-6.

Carpenter, M. W., and Donald R. Coustan. 1982. "Criteria for screening tests for gestational diabetes." *American Journal of Obstetrics & Gynecology* 144 (7):768-773.

Carr, D. B., and Steven Gabbe. 1998. "Gestational diabetes: detection, management, and implications." *Clinical Diabetes* 16 (1):4-12.

Catalano, P. M., Larraine Huston, Saeid B. Amini, and Satish C. Kalhan. 1999. "Longitudinal changes in glucose metabolism during pregnancy in obese women with normal glucose tolerance and gestational diabetes mellitus." *American Journal of Obstetrics and Gynecology* 180 (4):903-916.

Chiswick, C., R. M. Reynolds, F. Denison, A. J. Drake, S. Forbes, D. E. Newby, B. R. Walker, S. Quenby, S. Wray, A. Weeks, H. Lashen, A. Rodriguez, G. Murray, S. Whyte, and J. E. Norman. 2015. "Effect of metformin on maternal and fetal outcomes in obese pregnant women (EMPOWaR): a randomised, double-blind, placebo-controlled trial." *Lancet Diabetes Endocrinol* 3 (10):778-86. doi: 10.1016/s2213-8587(15)00219-3.

Corrado, F., R. D'Anna, G. Di Vieste, D. Giordano, B. Pintaudi, A. Santamaria, and A. Di Benedetto. 2011. "The effect of myoinositol supplementation on insulin resistance in patients with gestational diabetes." *Diabet Med* 28 (8):972-5. doi: 10.1111/j.1464-5491.2011.03284.x.

Costabile, L., and Unfer, V. (2017). "Treatment of gestational diabetes mellitus with myo-inositol: analyzing the cutting edge starting from a peculiar case." *Eur Rev Med Pharmacol Sci* 21 (2 Suppl):73-76.

Coustan, D. R. (2013). "Can a dietary supplement prevent gestational diabetes mellitus?" *Diabetes Care* 36 (4):777-779.

Crawford, T. J., Crowther, C. A., Alsweiler, J., Brown, J. (2015). "Antenatal dietary supplementation with myo-inositol in women during pregnancy for preventing gestational diabetes." *Cochrane Database Syst Rev* (12):Cd011507. doi: 10.1002/14651858.CD011507.pub2.

D'Anna, R., Di Benedetto, A., Scilipoti, A., Santamaria, A., Interdonato, M. L., Petrella, E., Neri, I., Pintaudi, B., Corrado, F., Facchinetti, F. (2015). "Myo-inositol supplementation for prevention of gestational diabetes in obese pregnant women: a randomized controlled trial." *Obstetrics & Gynecology* 126 (2):310-315.

D'anna, R., Di Benedetto, V., Rizzo, P., Raffone, E., Interdonato, M. L., Corrado, F., Di Benedetto, A. (2012). "Myo-inositol may prevent gestational diabetes in PCOS women." *Gynecological Endocrinology* 28 (6):440-442.

D'Anna, R., Scilipoti, A., Giordano, D., Caruso, C., Cannata, M. L., Interdonato, M. L., Corrado, F., Di Benedetto, A. (2013). "myo-Inositol Supplementation and Onset of Gestational Diabetes Mellitus in Pregnant Women with a Family History of Type 2 Diabetes: A prospective, randomized, placebo-controlled study." *Diabetes Care* 36 (4):854-857. doi: 10.2337/dc12-1371.

Dabelea, D. (2007). "The predisposition to obesity and diabetes in offspring of diabetic mothers." *Diabetes Care* 30 (Supplement 2):S169-S174.

Farren, M., Daly, N., McKeating, A., Kinsley, B., Turner, M. J., Daly, S. (2017). "The prevention of gestational diabetes mellitus with antenatal oral inositol supplementation: a randomized controlled trial." *Diabetes Care*:dc162449.

Feig, D. S., and Moses, R. G. (2011). "Metformin Therapy During Pregnancy." *Diabetes Care* 34 (10):2329.

Fraticelli, F., Celentano, C., Zecca, I. A. L., Di Vieste, G., Pintaudi, B., Liberati, M., Franzago, M., Di Nicola, M., Vitacolonna, E. (2018). "Effect of inositol stereoisomers at different dosages in gestational diabetes: an open-label, parallel, randomized controlled trial." *Acta Diabetologica*:1-8.

Gerli, S., Papaleo, E., Ferrari, A., Di Renzo, G. C. (2007). "Randomized, double blind placebo-controlled trial: effects of myo-inositol on ovarian function and metabolic factors in women with PCOS." *Eur Rev Med Pharmacol Sci* 11 (5):347-54.

Glueck, C. J., Pranikoff, J., Aregawi, D., Wang, P. (2008). "Prevention of gestational diabetes by metformin plus diet in patients with polycystic ovary syndrome." *Fertil Steril* 89 (3):625-34. doi: 10.1016/j.fertnstert.2007.03.036.

Glueck, C. J., Goldenberg, N., Streicher, P., Wang P. (2003). "Metformin and gestational diabetes." *Current Diabetes Reports* 3 (4):303-312. doi: 10.1007/s11892-003-0022-0.

Gray, S. G., McGuire, T. M., Cohen, N., Little, P. J. (2017). "The emerging role of metformin in gestational diabetes mellitus." *Diabetes Obes Metab* 19 (6):765-772. doi: 10.1111/dom.12893.

Group, Hapo Study Cooperative Research. (2008). "Hyperglycemia and adverse pregnancy outcomes." *New England Journal of Medicine* 358 (19):1991-2002.

Guo, X., Guo, S., Miao, Z., Li, Z., Zhang, H. (2017). "Myo-inositol lowers the risk of developing gestational diabetic mellitus in pregnancies: A systematic review and meta-analysis of randomized controlled trials with trial sequential analysis." *Journal of Diabetes and Its Complications*.

Haneda, M., Kikkawa, R., Arimura, T., Ebata, K., Togawa, M., Maeda, S., Sawada, T., Horide, N., Shigeta, Y. (1990). "Glucose inhibits myo-inositol uptake and reduces myo-inositol content in cultured rat glomerular mesangial cells." *Metabolism-Clinical and Experimental* 39 (1):40-45.

International Association of Diabetes and Panel Pregnancy Study Groups Consensus. (2010). "International association of diabetes and pregnancy study groups recommendations on the diagnosis and classification of hyperglycemia in pregnancy." *Diabetes Care* 33 (3):676-682.

Kennington, A. S., Hill, C. R., Craig, J., Bogardus, C., Raz, I., Ortmeyer, H. K., Hansen, B. C., Romero, G., Larner, J. (1990). "Low Urinary chiro-Inositol Excretion in Non-Insulin-Dependent Diabetes Mellitus."

New England Journal of Medicine 323 (6):373-378. doi: 10.1056/NEJM199008093230603.

Langer, O., Yogev, Y., Most, O., Xenakis, E. M. J. (2005). "Gestational diabetes: the consequences of not treating." *American Journal of Obstetrics and Gynecology* 192 (4):989-997.

Lee, H., Jang, H. C., Park, H. K., Cho, N. H. (2007). "Early manifestation of cardiovascular disease risk factors in offspring of mothers with previous history of gestational diabetes mellitus." *Diabetes Research and Clinical Practice* 78 (2):238-245.

Matarrelli, B., Vitacolonna, E., D'Angelo, M., Pavone, G., Mattei, P. A., Liberati, M., Celentano, M. (2013). "Effect of dietary myo-inositol supplementation in pregnancy on the incidence of maternal gestational diabetes mellitus and fetal outcomes: a randomized controlled trial." *J Matern Fetal Neonatal Med* 26 (10):967-72. doi: 10.3109/14767058.2013.766691.

Metzger, B. E., Buchanan, T. A., Coustan, D. R., De Leiva, A., Dunger, D. B., Hadden, D. R., Hod, M., Kitzmiller, J. L., Kjos, S. L., Oats. J. N. (2007). "Summary and recommendations of the fifth international workshop-conference on gestational diabetes mellitus." *Diabetes Care* 30 (Supplement 2):S251-S260.

Metzger, B. E., and Coustan, D. R. (1998). "Summary and recommendations of the fourth international workshop-conference on gestational diabetes mellitus." *Diabetes Care* 21:B161.

Nankervis, A., and Conn, J. (2013). "Gestational diabetes mellitus--negotiating the confusion." *Aust Fam Physician* 42 (8):528-31.

NICE, Women's National Collaborating Centre for Women and Health Children's. (2015). "National Institute for Health and Care Excellence: Clinical Guidelines." In *Diabetes in Pregnancy: Management of Diabetes and Its Complications from Preconception to the Postnatal Period*. London: National Institute for Health and Care Excellence (UK).

Pedersen, O. (1999). "Genetics of insulin resistance." *Experimental and Clinical Endocrinology & Diabetes* 107 (02):113-118.

Santamaria, A., Alibrandi, A., Di Benedetto, A., Pintaudi, B., Corrado, F., Facchinetti, F., D'Anna, R. (2018). "Clinical and metabolic outcomes in pregnant women at risk for gestational diabetes mellitus supplemented with myo-inositol: a secondary analysis from 3 RCTs." *American Journal of Obstetrics & Gynecology*.

Santamaria, A., Di Benedetto, A., Petrella, E., Pintaudi, B., Corrado, F., D'Anna, R., Neri, I., Facchinetti, F. (2016). "Myo-inositol may prevent gestational diabetes onset in overweight women: a randomized, controlled trial." *J Matern Fetal Neonatal Med* 29 (19):3234-7. doi: 10.3109/14767058.2015.1121478.

Shepherd, E., Gomersall, J. C., Tieu, J., Han, S., Crowther, C. A., Middleton, P. (2017). "Combined diet and exercise interventions for preventing gestational diabetes mellitus." *Cochrane Database Syst Rev* 11:Cd010443. doi: 10.1002/14651858.CD010443.pub3.

Tang, T., Lord, J. M., Norman, R. J., Yasmin, E., Balen, A. H. (2012). "Insulin-sensitising drugs (metformin, rosiglitazone, pioglitazone, D-chiro-inositol) for women with polycystic ovary syndrome, oligo amenorrhoea and subfertility." *Cochrane Database Syst Rev* (5):Cd003053. doi: 10.1002/14651858.CD003053.pub5.

Virkamäki, A., Ueki, K., Kahn, C. R. (1999). "Protein–protein interaction in insulin signaling and the molecular mechanisms of insulin resistance." *The Journal of Clinical Investigation* 103 (7):931-943.

Zhang, H., Lv, Y., Li, Z., Sun, L., Guo, W. (2018). "The efficacy of myo-inositol supplementation to prevent gestational diabetes onset: a meta-analysis of randomized controlled trials." *The Journal of Maternal-Fetal & Neonatal Medicine*: 1-7. doi: 10.1080/14767058.2018.1428303.

In: Inositols
Editor: Vittorio Unfer
ISBN: 978-1-53614-912-8

Chapter 6

INOSITOL RESISTANCE: A PROBLEM AND A SOLUTION

Zdravko Kamenov, MD, PhD, DMedSc and Antoaneta Gateva*, MD, PhD
Clinic of Endocrinology, University Hospital Alexandrovska,
Department of Internal Medicine,
Medical University Sofia, Sofia, Bulgaria

ABSTRACT

Myo-inositol (MI) and D-chiro-inositol (DCI) are involved in a number of biochemical pathways within oocytes having a role in oocyte maturation, fertilisation, implantation and postimplantation development. Some studies have demonstrated that MI treatment mainly in patients with polycystic ovary syndrome (PCOS) improved ovarian function and fertility, decreased the severity of hyperandrogenism including, acne and hirsutism, positively affected metabolic aspects and modulated various

* Corresponding Author's Email: tony_gateva@yahoo.com.

hormonal parameters. These parameters are deeply involved in the reproductive axis function and ovulation and thus MI treatment becomes a novel method to improve spontaneous ovulation or to induce ovulation. Despite the very good effect of MI on metabolic, hormonal and reprodutive parameters of PCOS patients, 20% to 40% of them could be resistant to this treatment. The reason for this resistance is still unclear but could be related to the state of obesity, insulin resistance and hyperandrogenemia or differences in compound bioavailability. Addition of α-lactalbumin, clomiphene citrate or rFSH can be a useful terapeutic alternative to overcome inositol resistance and achieve ovulation in these patients.

Keywords: myo-inositol, resistance, ovulation, PCOS

Introduction

Myo-inositol (MI) and D-chiro-inositol (DCI) are two of the nine different stereoisomers of inositol. They have important functions in the control of glucose homeostasis as second messengers involved in the signaling-transduction cascade of insulin (Huang et al. 1993, Larner et al. 1988). MI and DCI are also involved in a number of biochemical pathways within oocytes (Chiu et al. 2003, Matsuda et al. 2009) having a role in oocyte maturation, fertilisation, implantation and postimplantation development. DCI was found to be mainly involved in postreceptor insulin signaling (Iuorno and Nestler 2001, Nestler, Jakubowicz, and Iuorno 2000) and insulin-mediated androgen synthesis (Nestler and Unfer 2015), while MI regulates glucose uptake and follicle stimulating hormone (FSH) signaling (Nestler and Unfer 2015, Unfer et al. 2016).As MI was shown to be essential for proper oocyte maturation (Chiu et al. 2003) and direct correlation of MI concentration in the follicular fluid and high oocyte quality has been found (Chiu et al. 2002), its use in assisted reproduction technologies has drawn the interest of scientific community (Bevilacqua et al. 2015).

Inositols for Ovulation Induction – Effectiveness and Resistance

Some studies have demonstrated that MI treatment mainly in patients with polycystic ovary syndrome (PCOS) improved ovarian function and fertility (Papaleo et al. 2007, Papaleo et al. 2009, Raffone, Rizzo, and Benedetto 2010), decreased the severity of hyperandrogenism, acne and hirsutism (Ciotta et al. 2011, Minozzi, Nordio, and Pajalich 2013, Zacche et al. 2009), positively affected metabolic parameters and modulated various hormonal parameters deeply involved in the reproductive axis function and ovulation (Artini et al. 2013, Di Berardino et al. 2010) and thus it became a novel method to improve spontaneous ovulation (Genazzani et al. 2008, Gerli et al. 2007, Papaleo et al. 2007) or ovulation induction (Kamenov et al. 2015, Morgante et al. 2011, Papaleo et al. 2008). On the other hand MI treatment is safe and with very few side effects compared to other ovulation induction therapeutic options. Not all patients treated with inositols however ovulate and this failure can be regarded as *inositol resistance* (Kamenov et al. 2015). Based on the evidences in literature up to now, it can be estimated that the inositol resistance varies through different studies approximately from 20% to 40%.

Gerli et al. (2003) showed that ovulation frequency, defined by the luteal ratio, was significantly higher ($p<0.01$) in MI-treated group (23%) compared with placebo (13%). Estradiol (E2) concentration increased only in MI group during the first week of treatment inducing follicular maturation (Gerli, Mignosa, and Di Renzo 2003). Ovulation failed in 8 of the total 136 (5%) MI-treated patients during treatment, compared with 17 of 147 placebo-treated (11.5%). In another study by the same authors the ovulation frequency was similar and significantly higher in the MI treated group (25%) compared with placebo (15%), and the time to first ovulation was significantly shorter [24.5 d; 95% confidence interval (CI), 18, 31; compared with 40.5 d; 95% CI, 27, 54] (Gerli et al. 2007). Also this case ovulation failed in 8 of 45 (18%) MI-treated patients during treatment, compared with 17 of 47 placebo-treated (36%). The effect of MI on follicular maturation was rapid, because the E2 circulating concentration increased over the first week of treatment only in the MI group.

Raffone showed that 65% of MI treated patients restored spontaneous ovulation activity (30% of these obtained pregnancy), compared to 50% of metformin treated patients (18.3% of these obtained pregnancy) after a mean of 14.8 (±1.8) days and 16.7 (±2.5) days from the day 1 of the menstrual cycle, respectively (Raffone, Rizzo, and Benedetto 2010).

In another study ovulation was restored in 69.5% of women in MI group and 21% of placebo ($p = 0.001$). After treatment, the peak level of progesterone (P) was higher in MI patients (15.1 ± 2.2 ng/ml) compared to placebo (Costantino et al. 2009).

In a large observational study performed in 3602 infertile women with PCOS MI + folic acid treatment for a mean time of 10.2 weeks resulted in restoration of ovulation in 70% of women and 545 pregnancies (15.1% of all MI treated patients) (Regidor and Schindler 2016). A significant improvement of androgen levels and a rise in the progesterone values were observed during the treatment period.

In a study by Papaleo et al. (2007) 88% of patients with PCOS treated with MI restored at least one spontaneous menstrual cycle during 6 months, of whom 72% maintained normal ovulatory activity during the follow-up period activity, documented by follicular growth and increased serum progesterone concentrations in the luteal phase. Two out of the 22 women showed only a follicular development on ultrasound without progesterone elevation during weekly blood sampling, while two women did not have any further ovarian activity after the first cycle (Papaleo et al. 2007).

Compared to clomiphene citrate MI showed nonsignificant trend to lower resistance rate (30.6% vs 36.8%, $p = 0.62$), lower ovulation rate (69.4% vs 79.5% ($p = 0.31$) and higher pregnancy rate 33.3% vs 28.2% ($p = 0.13$). Among pregnancies, the multiple pregnancy rate was 18.1% in clomiphene group and 0% in the MI group (Papaleo et al. 2008).

In a study by Kamenov et al. (2015) MI monotherapy in PCOS patients with insulin resistance resulted in 61.7% ovulation rate (of those 37.9% became pregnant) during 3 spontaneous menstrual cycles (Kamenov et al. 2015).

MI supplementation also produced very good clinical results with a significant reduction in cancellation rate (0 vs. 40%) and the consequent improvement in clinical pregnancy rate (33.3% vs. 13.3%) in insulin-resistant patients with PCOS, undergoing gonadotropin ovulation induction using the low-dose step-down regime (Morgante et al. 2011).

In a very recent study following MI treatment 23 of 37 anovulatory women with PCOS (62%) ovulated, while 14 (38%) were resistant and did not ovulate (Montanino Oliva et al. 2018).

Summarizing the data, MI has been proven to induce the ovulation in most (up to 70%) of PCOS women, but still a part of them (around 30%) remain resistant.

Causes of Inositol Resistance

In most of the trials evaluating the rate of MI induced ovulation the differences in terms of hormonal and metabolic profile between responders and nonresponders were not assessed.

One study that compared 12 patients who responded to MI by establishing normal ovulation frequency (n = 6) and/or pregnancy (n = 6) with those patients who did not respond (less than three ovulations in 16 wk; n =9) showed that the two groups presented similar Body Mass Index (BMI), Waist to Hip Ratio (WHR), and circulating E2 and inhibin-B concentrations (Gerli et al. 2007). However, responders to MI treatment showed significantly lower testosterone levels (2.3 nmol/l vs. 3.4 nmol/l, respectively), higher Sex Hormone Binding Globulin (SHBG) (35.9 nmol/l vs. 25.8 nmol/l; $p < 0.05$), and thus lower free androgen index (6.9 vs. 11.6; $p = 0.01$). Fasting insulin or glucose concentrations or responses to the Oral Glucose Tolerance Test (OGTT) were not significantly different. The authors conclude that the least androgenic patients were more likely to respond with establishment of normal menstrual rhythm to MI treatment.

In the study by Kamenov et al. (2015) most of the women who ovulated or became pregnant with MI were normal weight or overweight, while most of the patients resistant to MI were obese. From the normal weight women,

73% became ovulating and 40% became pregnant. From the overweight women, 83% ovulated and 25% became pregnant and from the obese women 40% and 10% respectively. Compared to a normal weight woman, the obese had nearly the half probability to ovulate and a quarter the chance to become pregnant. Compared to non-obese women, the obese had half and one-third of the chance to become ovulating and pregnant, respectively. Generally, MI resistant women were of the same age as ovulating patients but were more obese with higher HOMA index on the third cycle during the treatment. On the other hand, patients who became pregnant during MI monotherapy had lower BMI at baseline (26.8 ± 5.8 versus 30.6 ± 7.6 kg/m^2, NS) and at third cycle (25.4 ± 5.7 *vs.* 30.2 ± 7.2 kg/m^2, $p < 0.01$) and lower HOMA index at baseline (4.0 ± 1.7 *vs.* 4.5 ± 2.6, NS) and at third cycle (2.3 ± 0.8 *vs.* 3.6 ± 2.1, $p < 0.05$) than those who did not achieve pregnancy.

In a recent study by Montanino et al. (2018) BMI did not change in MI responder and non-responder patients (the new means ± SD were 25.6 ± 1.7 and 25.8 ± 1.9kg/m^2, respectively, *vs.* 25.9 ± 1.2 kg/m^{2}at baseline), whereas the mean ± SD of HOMA Index decreased to 3.3 ± 1.1 in responders and was unchanged in MI-resistant subjects (5.44 ± 2.0), compared to 5.51 ± 1.9 at baseline. In MI resistant patients plasma levels of MI did not increase, raising the question about the role of MI bioavailability in non-responders. MI bioavailability is affected by many different factors, including intestinal absorption, transport from plasma into tissues, endogenous synthesis and catabolism, kidney excretion etc. MI homeostasis in cells and tissues is maintained at three different levels: intestinal absorption and renal excretion; carrier mediated transport from plasma/interstitial fluids into cells and endogenous synthesis and catabolism (Bizzarri et al. 2016). Different inositol transporters are responsible for uptake and intracellular distribution of inositol. According to their transport mechanism they can be divided into sodium ion coupled and proton coupled (Schneider 2015). Human inositol transporters have a role in various diseases such as Down syndrome, Alzheimer's disease and bipolar disorder, and for this reason they draw medical interest.

MI is consumed by humans mostly as phytic acid (inositol hexakisphosphate – InsP6). Bacterial phytases and phosphatases, homologous to mammalian InsP6 phosphatase, are mainly responsible for digesting dietary InsP6, releasing MI and phosphate that can further be actively absorbed by the mentioned transporters (Bizzarri et al. 2016). A new hypothesis about PCOS pathogenesis has emerged recently – dysbiosis of gut microbiota that can increase ovarian androgen synthesis, interfere with normal follicle development via triggering a chronic inflammatory response and insulin resistance (Liu et al. 2017, Tremellen and Pearce 2012). Gut microbiota and its metabolites have a role in inflammation pathway regulation, brain-gut peptide secretion and islet beta-cell proliferation (Barber et al. 2015, Liu et al. 2017, Vrieze et al. 2010). Significant differences in gut microbial species between PCOS and non-PCOS patients had been observed with increased levels of Bacteroides, Escherichia/Shigella and Streptococcus sp. and decreased of Akkermansia and Ruminococcaceae sp. (Liu et al. 2017). A correlation between these changes and the levels of ghrelin, testosterone and BMI was observed. Besides that a lower alpha diversity of gut microbiome that negatively correlated with hyperandrogenism, total testosterone and hirsutism was also observed in women with PCOS compared with healthy women(Torres et al. 2018). It is possible that gut disbiosis is also linked to the high prevalence of obesity seen in PCOS patients and that changes in gut microbiota composition and enzyme secretion could be responsible for impaired digestion and absorption of MI containing compounds thus decreasing its bioavalilability in PCOS women.

Taken together these data suggest that MI resistance is more likely in more obese, insulin resistant and hyperandrogenic women with PCOS. The exact mechanism of this resistance is however not clear. Having in mind the complex and multifactorial pathogenensis of PCOS, including different triggering mechanisms – central dysregulation of the hypothalamic "pacemaker" mechanisms, genetically determined and obesity potentiated insulin resistance, follicular quality and oocyte microenviorment, etc. it is understandable that different pathogenetic mechanisms will need different treatment. MI has been proven to affect several components of PCOS pathogenesis. Differences in MI bioavailability achieved during treatment however could be involved in the MI resistance.

Treatment Options in Inositol-Resistant Patients

In MI resistant patients, who fail to ovulate on monotherapy, a few different agents could be added to improve ovulation and pregnancy rate (clomiphene, recombinant follicle-stimulating hormone (rFSH), α-lactalbumin).

Clomiphene citrate is an estrogen receptor modulator that blocks the negative feedback mechanism resulting in increased secretion of FSH. Clomiphene is the first line treatment for ovulation induction in PCOS patients (Thessaloniki ESHRE/ASRM sponsored PCOS consensus workshop group. 2008). In a study by Kamenov et al. (2015) the MI resistant patients (38.3%) were treated with combination of MI and clomiphene citrate during next three cycles and on this combination 13 of the 18 patients (72.2%) ovulated and five (10.6%) did not achieve ovulation. Six out of the 13 ovulatory women (42.6% or 12.8% of all women) became pregnant and seven (53.8% or 14.9% of all women) did not. The authors concluded that in non-ovulating or nonpregnant patients after MI treatment a combination with clomiphene citrate could be useful to achieve the goal of ovulation/pregnancy.

In a study by Raffone et al. (2010) MI treated patients who did not achieve pregnancy (n=38) continued MI use and underwent ovulation induction with *rFSH* for a maximum of three attempts. A very low-dose protocol (37.5 U/day) beginning from the day two of menstrual cycle in a step-up regime was selected. Pregnancy occurred in a total of 11 women (28.9%). Eight of these pregnancies occurred in the MI resistant patients (n=17), whereas three in the group which had ovulation restored with MI alone.

α-lactalbumin is a protein found in milk (20-25% of whey) that has a role not only as a nutrient but as a factor for resorption of other nutrients such as vitamins and microelements. In a very recent study, 14 MI resistant

PCOS patients were treated with combination of 2 g MI plus 50 mg α-lactalbumin, twice a day, for three months. Among these 14 subjects, 12 (86%) ovulated (Montanino Oliva et al. 2018). Their MI plasma levels at the end of the treatment significantly improved compared to the baseline (35.0 ± 3.8 μmol/l vs. 17.0 ± 3.5 μmol/l,) and were similar to the patients who responded positively to the treatment with MI alone (38 ± 2.9 μmol/l). The addition of α-lactalbumin could play a beneficial role for MI bioavailability by changes in tight junctions permeability thus increasing plasma concentration in simultaneous administration (Montanino Oliva et al. 2018). *In-vivo* experiment in healthy subjects showed that although the peak concentration at 180 min was similar when MI was administered as monotherapy and in combination with α-lactalbumin, administration of MI and α-lactalbumin in a single dose lead to significantly higher plasma concentrations of MI (Monastra et al. 2018). *In-vitro* experiment by the same study group showed that MI absorption in Caco-2 cells was improved in the presence of digested α-lactalbumin because of changes in tight junction permeability (Monastra et al. 2018). In particular, MI passage through human intestinal Caco-2 cell line differentiated on permeable filters was increased almost 4.5-fold by the presence of 10 mg/ml α-lactalbumin peptides.

Another possible mechanism might involve the stimulation of glucagon-like peptide-2 (GLP-2) secretion from gut endocrine cells by α-lactalbumin hydrolysate which was observed in rats (Izumi et al. 2009) and was proven to enhance small intestine absorption (Kato, Yu, and Schwartz 1999). In specific conditions α-lactalbumin can also work as a suitable carrier to increase the passage of molecules across the intestinal barrier.

It is possible that α-lactalbumin could induce beneficial changes in gut microbiota, that is disregulated in PCOS patients in terms of species and the related number of strains. Imbalanced microbiota plays a role in chronic inflammation seen in PCOS and can hamper the absorption of a wide array of substances (Schippa and Conte 2014, Tremellen and Pearce 2012). α-lactalbumin has been patented as a probiotic agent (Maase 2002) and has been shown to improve the intestinal growth of specific bacterial groups (Wernimont et al. 2015).

At last, α-lactalbumin could have an independent role in improving chronic inflammation stage in PCOS by inhibiting type 2 cyclooxygenase (COX2) and decreasing IL-6 levels (Yamaguchi and Uchida 2007, Yamaguchi, Yoshida, and Uchida 2009) and its beneficial effect on glucose homeostasis (Yamaguchi and Takai 2014).

The gastrointestinal tolerance of α-lactalbumin was demonstrated in healthy infants, where the rate of gastrointestinal side effects of α-lactalbumin enriched formula were similar to those of human milk and much lower than standard formula (Davis et al. 2008).

CONCLUSION

Despite the beneficial effect of MI on metabolic, hormonal and reproductive parameters of PCOS patients, approximately 20% to 40% women could be resistant to this treatment. The reason for this resistance is still unclear but could be related to the state of obesity, insulin resistance and hyperandrogenemia or differences in compound bioavailability. Addition of α-lactalbumin, clomiphene citrate or rFSH can be a useful therapeutic alternative to overcome inositol resistance and achieve ovulation in these patients. Nevertheless, the safety and tolerance of these 3 compounds, which are respectively a nutrient and two drugs, need to be carefully considered. Indeed, α-lactalbumin has been included into the Generally Recognized As Safe (GRAS) food substances database (see U.S. Food and Drug Administration). Based on the clinical evidences this substance has been considered widely safe and well tolerated by infants and adults. For this reason, α-lactalbumin can be considered the ideal approach for counteracting MI resistance.

CONFLICT OF INTEREST

None.

REFERENCES

Artini, P. G., O. M. Di Berardino, F. Papini, A. D. Genazzani, G. Simi, M. Ruggiero, and V. Cela. 2013. "Endocrine and clinical effects of myo-inositol administration in polycystic ovary syndrome. A randomized study." *Gynecol Endocrinol* 29 (4):375-9. doi: 10.3109/09513590.2012.743020.

Barber, T. M., G. K. Dimitriadis, A. Andreou, and S. Franks. 2015. "Polycystic ovary syndrome: insight into pathogenesis and a common association with insulin resistance." *Clin Med (Lond)* 15 Suppl 6:s72-6. doi: 10.7861/clinmedicine.15-6-s72.

Bevilacqua, A., G. Carlomagno, S. Gerli, M. Montanino Oliva, P. Devroey, A. Lanzone, C. Soulange, F. Facchinetti, G. Carlo Di Renzo, M. Bizzarri, M. Hod, P. Cavalli, R. D'Anna, S. Benvenga, T. T. Chiu, and Z. A. Kamenov. 2015. "Results from the International Consensus Conference on myo-inositol and D-chiro-inositol in Obstetrics and Gynecology--assisted reproduction technology." *Gynecol Endocrinol* 31 (6):441-6. doi: 10.3109/09513590.2015.1006616.

Bizzarri, M., A. Fuso, S. Dinicola, A. Cucina, and A. Bevilacqua. 2016. "Pharmacodynamics and pharmacokinetics of inositol(s) in health and disease." *Expert Opin Drug Metab Toxicol* 12 (10):1181-96. doi: 10.1080/17425255.2016.1206887.

Chiu, T. T., M. S. Rogers, E. L. Law, C. M. Briton-Jones, L. P. Cheung, and C. J. Haines. 2002. "Follicular fluid and serum concentrations of myo-inositol in patients undergoing IVF: relationship with oocyte quality." *Hum Reprod* 17 (6):1591-6.

Chiu, Tony Tak Yu, Michael Scott Rogers, Christine Briton-Jones, and Christopher Haines. 2003. "Effects of myo-inositol on the in-vitro maturation and subsequent development of mouse oocytes." *Human Reproduction* 18 (2):408-416. doi: 10.1093/humrep/deg113.

Ciotta, L., M. Stracquadanio, I. Pagano, A. Carbonaro, M. Palumbo, and F. Gulino. 2011. "Effects of myo-inositol supplementation on oocyte's quality in PCOS patients: a double blind trial." *Eur Rev Med Pharmacol Sci* 15 (5):509-14.

Costantino, D., G. Minozzi, E. Minozzi, and C. Guaraldi. 2009. "Metabolic and hormonal effects of myo-inositol in women with polycystic ovary syndrome: a double-blind trial." *Eur Rev Med Pharmacol Sci* 13 (2):105-10.

Davis, A. M., B. J. Harris, E. L. Lien, K. Pramuk, and J. Trabulsi. 2008. "Alpha-lactalbumin-rich infant formula fed to healthy term infants in a multicenter study: plasma essential amino acids and gastrointestinal tolerance." *Eur J Clin Nutr* 62 (11):1294-301. doi: 10.1038/sj.ejcn.1602848.

Di Berardino, O.M., P. Monteleone, V. Valentino, M.Ruggiero, F.Papini, V.Cela, P.G.Artini, and A.R. Genazzani. 2010. "Myo-inositol administration in pcos patients after IVF." *14th World Congress of Gynecological Endocrinology, Florence, Italy.*

Genazzani, A. D., C. Lanzoni, F. Ricchieri, and V. M. Jasonni. 2008. "Myo-inositol administration positively affects hyperinsulinemia and hormonal parameters in overweight patients with polycystic ovary syndrome." *Gynecol Endocrinol* 24 (3):139-44. doi: 10.1080/09513590801893232.

Gerli, S., M. Mignosa, and G. C. Di Renzo. 2003. "Effects of inositol on ovarian function and metabolic factors in women with PCOS: a randomized double blind placebo-controlled trial." *Eur Rev Med Pharmacol Sci* 7 (6):151-9.

Gerli, S., E. Papaleo, A. Ferrari, and G. C. Di Renzo. 2007. "Randomized, double blind placebo-controlled trial: effects of myo-inositol on ovarian function and metabolic factors in women with PCOS." *Eur Rev Med Pharmacol Sci* 11 (5):347-54.

Huang, L. C., M. C. Fonteles, D. B. Houston, C. Zhang, and J. Larner. 1993. "Chiroinositol deficiency and insulin resistance. III. Acute glycogenic and hypoglycemic effects of two inositol phosphoglycan insulin mediators in normal and streptozotocin-diabetic rats in vivo." *Endocrinology* 132 (2):652-7. doi: 10.1210/endo.132.2.8425485.

Iuorno, M. J., and J. E. Nestler. 2001. "Insulin-lowering drugs in polycystic ovary syndrome." *Obstet Gynecol Clin North Am* 28 (1):153-64.

Izumi, H., S. Ishizuka, A. Inafune, T. Hira, K. Ozawa, T. Shimizu, M. Takase, and H. Hara. 2009. "alpha-Lactalbumin hydrolysate stimulates glucagon-like peptide-2 secretion and small intestinal growth in suckling rats." *J Nutr* 139 (7):1322-7. doi: 10.3945/jn.109.106401.

Kamenov, Z., G. Kolarov, A. Gateva, G. Carlomagno, and A. D. Genazzani. 2015. "Ovulation induction with myo-inositol alone and in combination with clomiphene citrate in polycystic ovarian syndrome patients with insulin resistance." *Gynecol Endocrinol* 31 (2):131-5. doi: 10.3109/09513590.2014.964640.

Kato, Y., D. Yu, and M. Z. Schwartz. 1999. "Glucagonlike peptide-2 enhances small intestinal absorptive function and mucosal mass in vivo." *J Pediatr Surg* 34 (1):18-20; discussion 20-1.

Larner, J., L. C. Huang, G. Tang, S. Suzuki, C. F. Schwartz, G. Romero, Z. Roulidis, K. Zeller, T. Y. Shen, A. S. Oswald, and et al. 1988. "Insulin mediators: structure and formation." *Cold Spring Harb Symp Quant Biol* 53 Pt 2:965-71.

Liu, R., C. Zhang, Y. Shi, F. Zhang, L. Li, X. Wang, Y. Ling, H. Fu, W. Dong, J. Shen, A. Reeves, A. S. Greenberg, L. Zhao, Y. Peng, and X. Ding. 2017. "Dysbiosis of Gut Microbiota Associated with Clinical Parameters in Polycystic Ovary Syndrome." *Front Microbiol* 8:324. doi: 10.3389/fmicb.2017.00324.

Maase, K.S.J.. 2002. Use of alpha-lactalbumin as prebiotic agent. In *WittopKoning THEPCBV*. Netherlands.

Matsuda, Miho, Koushirou Tsutsumi, Takashi Kanematsu, Kiyoko Fukami, Yoshihiro Terada, Tadaomi Takenawa, Keiichi I. Nakayama, and Masato Hirata. 2009. "Involvement of Phospholipase C-Related Inactive Protein in the Mouse Reproductive System Through the Regulation of Gonadotropin Levels1." *Biology of Reproduction* 81 (4):681-689. doi: 10.1095/biolreprod.109.076760.

Minozzi, M., M. Nordio, and R. Pajalich. 2013. "The Combined therapy myo-inositol plus D-Chiro-inositol, in a physiological ratio, reduces the cardiovascular risk by improving the lipid profile in PCOS patients." *Eur Rev Med Pharmacol Sci* 17 (4):537-40.

Monastra, G., S. Ferruzza, Y. Sambuy, G. Ranaldi, and D. Ferrari. 2018. "Alpha-lactalbumin effect on myo-inositol intestinal absorption: in vivo and in vitro." *Curr Drug Deliv*. doi: 10.2174/1567201815666180509102641.

Montanino Oliva, M., G. Buonomo, M. Calcagno, and V. Unfer. 2018. "Effects of myo-inositol plus alpha-lactalbumin in myo-inositol-resistant PCOS women." *J Ovarian Res* 11 (1):38. doi: 10.1186/s13048-018-0411-2.

Morgante, G., R. Orvieto, A. Di Sabatino, M. C. Musacchio, and V. De Leo. 2011. "The role of inositol supplementation in patients with polycystic ovary syndrome, with insulin resistance, undergoing the low-dose gonadotropin ovulation induction regimen." *Fertil Steril* 95 (8):2642-4. doi: 10.1016/j.fertnstert.2011.01.035.

Nestler, J. E., D. J. Jakubowicz, and M. J. Iuorno. 2000. "Role of inositolphosphoglycan mediators of insulin action in the polycystic ovary syndrome." *J Pediatr Endocrinol Metab* 13 Suppl 5:1295-8.

Nestler, J. E., and V. Unfer. 2015. "Reflections on inositol(s) for PCOS therapy: steps toward success." *Gynecol Endocrinol* 31 (7):501-5. doi: 10.3109/09513590.2015.1054802.

Papaleo, E., L. De Santis, J. Baillargeon, M. Zacche, F. Fusi, C. Brigante, and A.Ferrari. 2008. "Comparison of myo-inositol plus folicacid vs clomiphene citrate for first line treatment in womenwithpolycysticovary syndrome." *24th Annual Meeting of ESHRE*, Barcelona, Spain.

Papaleo, E., V. Unfer, J. P. Baillargeon, L. De Santis, F. Fusi, C. Brigante, G. Marelli, I. Cino, A. Redaelli, and A. Ferrari. 2007. "Myo-inositol in patients with polycystic ovary syndrome: a novel method for ovulation induction." *Gynecol Endocrinol* 23 (12):700-3. doi: 10.1080/09513590701672405.

Papaleo, E., V. Unfer, J. P. Baillargeon, F. Fusi, F. Occhi, and L. De Santis. 2009. "Myo-inositol may improve oocyte quality in intracytoplasmic sperm injection cycles. A prospective, controlled, randomized trial." *Fertil Steril* 91 (5):1750-4. doi: 10.1016/j.fertnstert.2008.01.088.

Raffone, E., P. Rizzo, and V. Benedetto. 2010. "Insulin sensitiser agents alone and in co-treatment with r-FSH for ovulation induction in PCOS women." *Gynecol Endocrinol* 26 (4):275-80. doi: 10.3109/09513590903366996.

Regidor, P. A., and A. E. Schindler. 2016. "Myoinositol as a Safe and Alternative Approach in the Treatment of Infertile PCOS Women: A German Observational Study." *Int J Endocrinol* 2016:9537632. doi: 10.1155/2016/9537632.

Schippa, S., and M. P. Conte. 2014. "Dysbiotic events in gut microbiota: impact on human health." *Nutrients* 6 (12):5786-805. doi: 10.3390/nu6125786.

Schneider, Sabine. 2015. "Inositol transport proteins." *FEBS Letters* 589 (10):1049-1058. doi: https://doi.org/10.1016/j.febslet.2015.03.012.

Torres, P. J., M. Siakowska, B. Banaszewska, L. Pawelczyk, A. J. Duleba, S. T. Kelley, and V. G. Thackray. 2018. "Gut Microbial Diversity in Women with Polycystic Ovary Syndrome Correlates with Hyperandrogenism." *J Clin Endocrinol Metab* 103 (4):1502-1511. doi: 10.1210/jc.2017-02153.

Tremellen, Kelton, and Karma Pearce. 2012. *Dysbiosis of Gut Microbiota (DOGMA) - A novel theory for the development of Polycystic Ovarian Syndrome*. Vol. 79.

Unfer, Vittorio, John E. Nestler, Zdravko A. Kamenov, Nikos Prapas, and Fabio Facchinetti. 2016. "Effects of Inositol(s) in Women with PCOS: A Systematic Review of Randomized Controlled Trials." *International Journal of Endocrinology* 2016:12. doi: 10.1155/2016/1849162.

Vrieze, A., F. Holleman, E. G. Zoetendal, W. M. de Vos, J. B. L. Hoekstra, and M. Nieuwdorp. 2010. "The environment within: how gut microbiota may influence metabolism and body composition." *Diabetologia* 53 (4):606-613. doi: 10.1007/s00125-010-1662-7.

Wernimont, Susan, Robert Northington, Martin J. Kullen, Manjiang Yao, and Jodi Bettler. 2015. "Effect of an α-Lactalbumin-Enriched Infant Formula Supplemented With Oligofructose on Fecal Microbiota, Stool Characteristics, and Hydration Status: A Randomized, Double-Blind, Controlled Trial." *Clinical Pediatrics* 54 (4):359-370. doi: 10.1177/0009922814553433.

Yamaguchi, M., and M. Uchida. 2007. "Alpha-lactalbumin suppresses interleukin-6 release after intestinal ischemia/reperfusion via nitric oxide in rats." *Inflammopharmacology* 15 (1):43-7. doi: 10.1007/s10787-006-1558-9.

Yamaguchi, M., K. Yoshida, and M. Uchida. 2009. "Novel functions of bovine milk-derived alpha-lactalbumin: anti-nociceptive and anti-inflammatory activity caused by inhibiting cyclooxygenase-2 and phospholipase A2." *Biol Pharm Bull* 32 (3):366-71.

Yamaguchi, Makoto, and Shoko Takai. 2014. "Chronic Administration of Bovine Milk-Derived α-Lactalbumin Improves Glucose Tolerance <i>via</i> Enhancement of Adiponectin in Goto–Kakizaki Rats with Type 2 Diabetes." *Biological and Pharmaceutical Bulletin* 37 (3):404-408. doi: 10.1248/bpb.b13-00762.

Zacche, M. M., L. Caputo, S. Filippis, G. Zacche, M. Dindelli, and A. Ferrari. 2009. "Efficacy of myo-inositol in the treatment of cutaneous disorders in young women with polycystic ovary syndrome." *Gynecol Endocrinol* 25 (8):508-13. doi: 10.1080/09513590903015544.

In: Inositols
Editor: Vittorio Unfer
ISBN: 978-1-53614-912-8

Chapter 7

INOSITOLS VS. METFORMIN: COMPARISON BETWEEN INSULIN SENSITIZERS

Pedro-Antonio Regidor*, PhD
Exeltis Healthcare, Ismaning, Germany

ABSTRACT

Polycystic Ovary Syndrome (PCOS) is a disease that causes irregular bleedings, chronic anovulation, androgen excess and a typical ovarian ultrasound feature. It is the most common cause of infertility affecting between 5% -10% of women during their reproductive age. Several studies have shown how the improvement of insulin sensitivity is beneficial in the treatment of complex disorder like PCOS. For this reason I will discuss thoroughly the importance of insulin sensitizers, such as Inositol and Metformine.

Keywords: inositol, myo-inositol, d-chiro-inositol, metformine, insulin sensitizers, polycystic ovary syndrome

---

* Corresponding Author's Email: pedro-antonio.regidor@exeltis.com.

INTRODUCTION

Polycystic Ovary Syndrome (PCOS) is a disease that causes irregular bleedings, chronic anovulation, androgen excess and a typical ovarian ultrasound feature (Ehrmann 2005). It is the most common cause of infertility affecting between 5% -10% of women during their reproductive age (Homburg 1996). The PCOS etiopathology is not clear, but most probably a strong genetic cause, influenced by gestational environment and lifestyle, seems to be the key factor. The European Society of Human reproduction and Embryology and the American Society for reproductive Medicine defined at a meeting in Rotterdam 2003 the criteria for the definition of this disease (Rotterdam 2004). To reach a general agreement on diagnostic criteria many investigations have focused, independently of the above-mentioned disorders on the impaired glucose tolerance, which affects 30 – 40% of women with PCOS (Ehrmann et al. 1999) and on insulin resistance. Hyperinsulinemia due to insulin resistance occurs in up to 80% of women with PCOS and central obesity as well as in 30 – 40% of lean women diagnosed with this syndrome (Ciampelli et al. 1999, Genazzani et al. 2004, Genazzani et al. 2008).

The related hyperinsulinemia could induce an excess of androgens production in PCOS women through two different ways: first one is the direct stimulation of ovaries to produce androgens, the other one is the reduction of sex hormone binding globulin (SHBG) serum levels (Croze and Soulage 2013).

Due to the key role of insulin in the syndrome etiopathology, since many years insulin sensitizers such as metformin, pioglitazone or troglitazone have been considered as possible therapeutic options. Metformin has been used in the last time on patients with a hyperinsulinemic status for the improvement of ovarian dysfunction with consecutive anovulation, irregular menstrual cycles, and infertility problems (Baillargeon, Iuorno, and Nestler 2003, Genazzani et al. 2004). Nevertheless Metformin, when used in the therapeutically dose range, has shown to have several side effects such as flatulence, diarrhea, and nausea, so that many patients are unable to use this treatment option in gynecology for a longer period (Kim et al. 2012, Strugaru et al. 2013).

In addition, to the common use of metformin and other insulin sensitizer agents for the treatment of PCOS, in the recent years other therapeutic alternatives have been investigated, especially myo-inositol (MI).

INOSITOL

The substance inositol is a chemical compound with the formula C6H12O6 or (-CHOH-)6, a six-fold alcohol (polyol) of cyclohexane with five equatorial and one axial hydroxyl group. It is widely found in nature. Nine different stereoisomer forms have been described, but MI is the most common found in nature. In fact, MI is very often found in many plants and in tissues of animals. The second most common form is D-chiro-inositol (DCI). It is important to distinguish between the lecithin formulation that is bioavailable for the human and the phytate formulation of corns that are not bioavailable. Food with the highest concentration of MI are fruits, beans, corns and nuts (Clements and Darnell 1980).

Inositol was defined in the past as "myometrial sugar," but it is indeed not a substance belonging to the carbohydrate group. Defining inositol as a vitamin B is also being discussed with controversy as inositol is not an essential substance and it can be produced in human cells from glucose (Reynolds 1982). In fact, several studies have proved that the inositol molecule is directly involved in the insulin cellular signaling.

Regarding PCOS, several studies have shown that one of the mechanisms of insulin deficiency has its rise from the inositolphosphoglycan (IPG) mediator and that a deficiency of inositol in the IPGs is responsible for insulin resistance. It has been demonstrated that the administration of DCI (intracellularly converted from MI) reduces the insulin resistance (Baillargeon et al. 2008, Hooper 1997).

Studies have suggested that an impairment of the insulin pathway could be due to a defect in the IPGs second messenger (Asplin, Galasko, and Larner 1993, Kennington et al. 1990). IPGs play a role in activating enzymes that control glucose metabolism (Baillargeon et al. 2008, Cohen 2006). In PCOS women, a defect in tissue availability or altered metabolism of inositol or IPGs mediators may contribute to insulin resistance (Baillargeon et al. 2006). Previous studies have demonstrated that MI is able to restore spontaneous ovarian activity in PCOS women and consequently fertility in many of these cases (Papaleo et al. 2007).

Nevertheless, many of these PCOS women require techniques of assisted reproduction to achieve a pregnancy. However, more than 60% of *in vitro* fertilization (IVF) cycles do not result in a pregnancy and poor oocyte quality is the main cause of fertilization failure (Serhal et al. 1997). Therefore, assisted reproductive techniques nowadays focus on obtaining high quality oocytes rather than high numbers of oocytes and embryos (Macklon and Fauser 2003). In IVF techniques, the supplementation with MI is positively correlated to a meiotic progression of mouse germinal vesicle oocytes, enhancing intracellular Ca^{2+} oscillations (Chiu et al. 2002). In follicular human fluids, higher concentrations of MI represent a marker of good quality oocytes (Chiu et al. 2003).

If at the end MI or DCI have a better effect on the quality of the oocytes in IVF cycles must be elucidated. The paradox theory published and discussed by Nestler and Carlomagno (Carlomagno, Unfer, and Roseff 2011, Nestler and Unfer 2015) suggest that DCI in not physiological high dosages have a negative impact on the quality of oocytes of PCOS women, as the ovarian epimerase function is not altered in PCOS patients so that the MI levels in the follicular fluids remain low if only DCI is supplemented. The Consensus Conference on MI and DCI postulated that the future ideal inositol supplementation should therefore contain a ratio of 40:1 between MI and DCI (Facchinetti et al. 2015).

The approach of MI with 3 mg melatonin is also a way in the possible improvement of oocyte quality. Rizzo et al. and Unfer et al. could obtain oocytes with a better quality when the PCOS women were treated in the combination with MI 4 g + 400 μg folic acid + 3 mg melatonin per day in comparison to formulations without melatonin (Rizzo, Raffone, and Benedetto 2010, Unfer et al. 2011).

Studies report also a very good safety profile of the molecule, even when administered up to 12 g/day, where only mild gastrointestinal side effects have been reported (Carlomagno and Unfer 2011).

METFORMIN AND OTHER INSULIN SENSITIZERS

Metformin

Metformin is a synthetically derived biguanide, off-label used in the management of dysmetabolic disorders and insulin resistance in PCOS.

The effects of metformin on glucose metabolism seem to be secondary to its actions on the mitochondrial respiratory chain, inhibiting the mitochondrial respiratory complex I (Doran and Halestrap 2000, El-Mir et al. 2000). Therefore, it leads to a reduction in ATP production and oxidative phosphorylation, resulting in a higher AMP/ATP ratio which in turn inhibits gluconeogenesis and modulates AMPK. AMPK activation by metformin induces fatty acid oxidation, reduces lipid synthesis, and inhibits gluconeogenesis (Li et al. 2011, McGarry and Brown 1997).

Among the pharmacological therapies to treat PCOS, insulin-sensitizing agents are, as exposed before, fundamental to correct the underlying metabolic abnormalities. Metformin has of course also its important role in this disease. Both metformin and hormonal contraceptives (HCs) are very often used in adolescents with PCOS (Legro et al. 2013). Metformin, the primary insulin-sensitizing agent, is commonly used alone or in a low-dose combination with flutamide, or with both flutamide and pioglitazone (PioFluMet) (Díaz et al. 2012) as the PCOS is linked to insulin resistance which results in a compensatory increase in insulin secretion by the islet cells of the pancreas to maintain normal glucose homeostasis (Azziz et al. 2009). As also described above, this secondary hyperinsulinemia leads to many PCOS phenotypic features, such as ovarian hyperandrogenism and acanthosis nigricans. It decreases the production of SHBG. Insulin resistance further leads to metabolic complications including type 2 diabetes mellitus (T2DM), dyslipidemia, and metabolic syndrome. Moreover, obesity in

PCOS further worsens the metabolic parameters in PCOS women (Azziz et al. 2009). Therefor some authors recommend HCs with progestogens with an anti-androgenetic partial activity as first-line therapy for PCOS (Legro et al. 2013). The guidelines recommend metformin in those patients with PCOS who have T2DM or impaired glucose tolerance and failed lifestyle modification. For women with PCOS with menstrual irregularity who cannot take or do not tolerate HCs, metformin is suggested as a second-line therapy (Legro et al. 2013).

Metformin appears to have a direct effect on steroidogenesis in the ovaries regardless of its influence on insulin sensitivity. Metformin also decreases LH-stimulated testosterone secretion soon after use (Kurzthaler et al. 2014). However, the exact mechanism of action in PCOS is still not completely understood. Kurzthaler found no effect of metformin on body weight, insulin sensitivity and metabolic indices such as low-density lipoproteins (LDL), high-density lipoproteins (HDL), and triglycerides following three months of use. However, a significant decline in serum testosterone was observed after a relatively short course of treatment (Kurzthaler et al. 2014). Likewise, when adolescents with hyperandrogenic type 1 diabetes mellitus (T1DM) were treated with metformin, serum androgens decreased significantly, but other parameters of PCOS like hirsutism, ovulation, and metabolic indices did not alter significantly (Codner et al. 2013). Therefore, until now, metformin does not seem to have a beneficial role in treating hirsutism, acne, and infertility (Legro et al. 2013). The Endocrine Society clinical practice guidelines suggest against the use of metformin as a first-line treatment of skin manifestations, hirsutism, for the prevention of pregnancy complications, or for the treatment of obesity (Legro et al. 2013).

However, Naderpoor, et al. recently proposed that metformin treatment considerably improves body mass index (BMI), serum lipids, and glucose homeostasis. A combination of lifestyle and metformin is more beneficial than lifestyle alone in reducing BMI and adipose tissue levels. It also regulates the menstrual cycle in women with PCOS (Naderpoor et al. 2015). Many of the existing studies on the role of metformin in PCOS have limitations based on small sample sizes, bias risk, and short durations (Naderpoor et al. 2015).

Pioglitazone

Insulin-sensitizing agents are the initial treatment option in PCOS and pioglitazone is one of them. Treatment with pioglitazone is known to improve menstrual irregularities and hirsutism in PCOS. It also modifies other parameters linked to a higher risk of T2DM and cardiovascular diseases. Pioglitazone 30 mg/day leads to an increase in adiponectin with a reduction of insulin resistance. Fibrinogen and C-reactive protein (CRP) levels are also decreased (Stabile et al. 2014). Pioglitazone significantly improves endocrine and metabolic parameters in women with PCOS, and it can be a suitable alternative to metformin in women who are unable to take or tolerate metformin (Shahebrahimi et al. 2016). However, its use has been limited to patients with diabetes because of the associated cancer risk of thiazolidinediones and the eventual weight gain. The international guidelines do not favor thiazolidinediones because they do not have an overall favorable risk-benefit ratio (Legro et al. 2013).

DISCUSSION

PCOS is one of the most common endocrine disorders affecting women. Insulin resistance and hyperinsulinemia are often found in a high proportion of women with PCOS. A defect in insulin action has been postulated, possibly because of a deficiency of DCI, which is a component of inositol phosphoglycans. Insulin-lowering medications, particularly MI, represent novel therapies for restoring spontaneous ovulation, with a potential positive effect also on human oocyte meiotic maturation. This therapy appears to influence steroidogenesis directly, reducing the androgen production in theca cells. It was shown that inositol administration increases the action of insulin in patients with PCOS, thereby improving ovulatory function and decreasing serum testosterone concentration (Baillargeon et al. 2006, Gerli, Mignosa, and Di Renzo 2003, Iuorno et al. 2002, Nestler et al. 1999, Unfer et al. 2016).

Despite clear limitations of observational studies, the presented data are reliable, since a wide range of patients was analyzed. This study could show that a new treatment option for patients with a PCOS and infertility is available. Seventy% of the patients restored ovulation after the treatment. Furthermore, the achieved pregnancy rates are at least in an equivalent or even superior range than those reported using the insulin sensitizer metformin. Karimzadeh et al. (Karimzadeh and Javedani 2010) described a pregnancy rate of 14.4% in a cohort of 90 women and Legro et al. (Legro et al. 2007) of 12.3% in a cohort of 75 women with PCOS.

Another important evidence is also related to the difference of MI and metformin in terms of safety profile and compliance for patients. In patients under metformin side effects have been commonly reported, from mild up to sever gastrointestinal side effects, such as abdominal pain, nausea, diarrhea. Only in rare cases, very severe side effects as lactic acidosis have been found. On the other side, MI seems to be a safe and well-tolerated approach, anyhow able to give similar results of metformin in terms of clinical efficacy.

Many studies have demonstrated in the last months that an improvement in the rates of ovulation and regularization of menstrual cycles was obtained by the combined use of 4 g MI with 400 μg folic acid per day. Gerli et al. (Gerli et al. 2007) could show in a prospective study that the group of patients receiving MI + folic acid experienced in 82% of the cases an ovulation, whereas this was only observed in 63% of the cases in the group of patients, which received a placebo. By the same way 70% of the patients of MI group developed regular menstrual cycles after 16 weeks of treatment, whereas only 13% of the women did it in the placebo group.

In a study of Raffone et al. (Raffone, Rizzo, and Benedetto 2010), where a comparison between the administration of MI (2 x 2000 mg + 200 μg per day) and metformin (1500 mg per day) in women with a PCO syndrome was performed, it could be shown that the number of pregnancies was clearly higher in the MI group than in the metformin group of patients.

Some other studies upon others have shown the efficacy of MI in the improvement of the fertility of PCOS patients due to its improvement of the insulin resistance of these women (Morgante et al. 2011, Raffone, Rizzo, and Benedetto 2010, Sun et al. 2002, Genazzani et al. 2012).

Regarding the outcome of IVF cycles in women with a history of a PCOS Papaleo et al. could show that in patients with PCOS the treatment with MI and folic acid, but not folic acid alone, reduced germinal vesicles and degenerated oocytes at ovum pick-up without compromising total number of retrieved oocytes (Papaleo et al. 2009). By the same way the amount of stimulation days was, as in our study, shorter in the MI treated women showing a faster response of the ovarian follicles to FSH stimulation due to the MI effects.

On the other side PCOS women have an increased risk of hyper stimulation syndrome (Battaglia et al. 2004). High levels of serum ovarian androgens are associated to a production of elevated serum E2 levels after gonadotropin ovarian stimulation. The study of Papaleo (2009) showed that PCOS patients treated with MI and gonadotropin had a significant reduction in E2 levels after hGC administration (Papaleo et al. 2009). This was related also to the lower number of IVF cycles cancelled because of high E2 levels (sign of hyper stimulation syndrome).

In addition to this, MI is an important constituent of follicular fluid, playing a key role in both nuclear and cytoplasmic oocyte development. In fact, supplementation with MI in the IVF technique is positively associated to meiotic progression of mouse germinal vesicle oocytes, enhancing intracellular Ca^2 oscillation (Battaglia et al. 2004). In human follicular fluids, higher concentrations of MI provide a marker of good-quality oocytes (Papaleo et al. 2009, Unfer et al. 2016, Unfer et al. 2011).

Beside the increased ratio follicles/retrieved oocytes and the higher fertilization rate in the group of women that used MI, a more important result was the increased number of top-quality (score 1 versus 2) embryos in the MI group. These data suggest that, besides increasing the fertilization rate, MI supplementation has also an effect on the overall quality of the oocyte pool.

Many studies have been performed that show that the treatment with MI + folic acid in the classical dosage (2 x 2000 mg MI+200 µg folic acid per day) leads to significant positive changes of metabolic and hormonal parameters. Constantino et al. (59) could show in a double-blinded, placebo-controlled study that MI lead to a statistically significant improvement of the blood pressure, triglycerides, cholesterol, glucose and insulin values after a 75 mg oral glucose tolerance test. These improvements were achieved after a treatment period of 16 weeks. The evaluated hormonal values showed a significant decrease of the total and free testosterone serum levels and at the same time the progesterone levels, as a marker of ovulation, experienced a significant rise in the group that received MI. This could show that MI did not only lead to positive changes in metabolic parameters but also to a reduction of elevated androgenic values and subsequently to an improvement of skin problems such as acne or hirsutism.

These data can be supported by our own data as a rise of progesterone from a value of 2.1 ng/ml to a value of 12.3 ng/ml could be observed. By the same time a reduction in the levels of testosterone (from 96.6 ng/ml to 43.3 ng/dl) and free testosterone (from 1.2 ng/ml to 0.35 ng/ml) could also be observed.

This confirms that MI is not only an effective alternative in the treatment of PCOS patients but also a secure one as no side effects could be observed in the standard dosage. This is on the other side relevant as the compliance of the use rises resulting in better outcomes in the management of ovulation, hyperandrogenism and metabolic parameters on patients with a PCOS.

When comparing a combination of both substances like done by Fruzzetti et al. to evaluate clinical and metabolic features in women with a PCOS it could be shown that there were no significant differences in the outcome analyses (Fruzzetti et al. 2017). The use of 4000 mg MI per day was equal to the use of 1500 mg metformin per day over a 6-month period.

Conclusion

As a result, both substances have its rational place in the management of women with PCOS.

Even though, additional investigations on larger number of patients are needed to further characterize the impact of both substances on oocyte follicular development and oocyte maturation, and its implication in stimulation and pregnancy outcomes in IVF procedures.

References

Asplin, I., G. Galasko, and J. Larner. 1993. "chiro-inositol deficiency and insulin resistance: a comparison of the chiro-inositol- and the myo-inositol-containing insulin mediators isolated from urine, hemodialysate, and muscle of control and type II diabetic subjects." *Proc Natl Acad Sci USA* 90 (13):5924-8.

Azziz, R., E. Carmina, D. Dewailly, E. Diamanti-Kandarakis, H. F. Escobar-Morreale, W. Futterweit, O. E. Janssen, R. S. Legro, R. J. Norman, A. E. Taylor, and S. F. Witchel. 2009. "The Androgen Excess and PCOS Society criteria for the polycystic ovary syndrome: the complete task force report." *Fertil Steril* 91 (2):456-88. doi: 10.1016/j.fertnstert.2008.06.035.

Baillargeon, J. P., E. Diamanti-Kandarakis, R. E. Ostlund, Jr., T. Apridonidze, M. J. Iuorno, and J. E. Nestler. 2006. "Altered D-chiro-inositol urinary clearance in women with polycystic ovary syndrome." *Diabetes Care* 29 (2):300-5.

Baillargeon, J. P., M. J. Iuorno, and J. E. Nestler. 2003. "Insulin sensitizers for polycystic ovary syndrome." *Clin Obstet Gynecol* 46 (2):325-40.

Baillargeon, J.-P., J. E. Nestler, R. E. Ostlund, T. Apridonidze, and E. Diamanti-Kandarakis. 2008. "Greek hyperinsulinemic women, with or without polycystic ovary syndrome, display altered inositols metabolism." *Human Reproduction* 23 (6):1439-1446.

Battaglia, C., F. Mancini, N. Persico, V. Zaccaria, and D. de Aloysio. 2004. "Ultrasound evaluation of PCO, PCOS and OHSS." *Reproductive Biomedicine Online* 9 (6):614-619.

Carlomagno, G., and V. Unfer. 2011. "Inositol safety: clinical evidences." *Eur Rev Med Pharmacol Sci* 15 (8):931-6.

Carlomagno, G., V. Unfer, and S. Roseff. 2011. "The D-chiro-inositol paradox in the ovary." *Fertil Steril* 95 (8):2515-6. doi: 10.1016/j.fertnstert.2011.05.027.

Chiu, T. T., M. S. Rogers, E. L. Law, C. M. Briton-Jones, L. P. Cheung, and C. J. Haines. 2002. "Follicular fluid and serum concentrations of myo-inositol in patients undergoing IVF: relationship with oocyte quality." *Hum Reprod* 17 (6):1591-6.

Chiu, T., T. Yu, M. S. Rogers, C. Briton- Jones, and C. Haines. 2003. "Effects of myo- inositol on the *in vitro* maturation and subsequent development of mouse oocytes." *Human Reproduction* 18 (2):408-416. doi: 10.1093/humrep/deg113.

Ciampelli, M., A. M. Fulghesu, F. Cucinelli, V. Pavone, E. Ronsisvalle, M. Guido, A. Caruso, and A. Lanzone. 1999. "Impact of insulin and body mass index on metabolic and endocrine variables in polycystic ovary syndrome." *Metabolism-Clinical and Experimental* 48 (2):167-172.

Clements, Jr R. S., and B. Darnell. 1980. "Myo-inositol content of common foods: development of a high-myo-inositol diet." *The American Journal of Clinical Nutrition* 33 (9):1954-1967. doi: 10.1093/ajcn/33.9.1954.

Codner, E., G. Iñíguez, P. López, V. Mujica, F. C. Eyzaguirre, S. Asenjo, I. Torrealba, and F. Cassorla. 2013. "Metformin for the treatment of hyperandrogenism in adolescents with type 1 diabetes mellitus." *Hormone Research in Paediatrics* 80 (5):343-349.

Cohen, P.. 2006. "The twentieth century struggle to decipher insulin signalling." *Nature Reviews Molecular Cell Biology* 7 (11):867.

Croze, M. L., and C. O. Soulage. 2013. "Potential role and therapeutic interests of myo-inositol in metabolic diseases." *Biochimie* 95 (10):1811-27. doi: 10.1016/j.biochi.2013.05.011.

Díaz, M., M. R. Chacon, A. Lopez-Bermejo, E. Maymo-Masip, C. Salvador, J. Vendrell, F. de Zegher, and L. Ibanez. 2012. "Ethinyl estradiolcyproterone acetate versus low-dose pioglitazone-flutamide-metformin for adolescent girls with androgen excess: divergent effects on CD163, TWEAK receptor, ANGPTL4, and LEPTIN expression in subcutaneous adipose tissue." *The Journal of Clinical Endocrinology & Metabolism* 97 (10):3630-3638.

Doran, E., and A. P. Halestrap. 2000. "Evidence that metformin exerts its anti-diabetic effects through inhibition of complex 1 of the mitochondrial respiratory chain." *Biochemical Journal* 348 (3):607-614.

Ehrmann, D. A., R. B. Barnes, R. L. Rosenfield, M. K. Cavaghan, and J. Imperial. 1999. "Prevalence of impaired glucose tolerance and diabetes in women with polycystic ovary syndrome." *Diabetes Care* 22 (1):141-6.

Ehrmann, David A. 2005. "Polycystic ovary syndrome." *New England Journal of Medicine* 352 (12):1223-1236.

El-Mir, M.-Y., V. Nogueira, E. Fontaine, N. Avéret, M. Rigoulet, and X. Leverve. 2000. "Dimethylbiguanide inhibits cell respiration via an indirect effect targeted on the respiratory chain complex I." *Journal of Biological Chemistry* 275 (1):223-228.

Facchinetti, F., M. Bizzarri, S. Benvenga, R. D'Anna, A. Lanzone, C. Soulage, G. C. Di Renzo, M. Hod, P. Cavalli, T. T. Chiu, Z. A. Kamenov, A. Bevilacqua, G. Carlomagno, S. Gerli, M. M. Oliva, and P. Devroey. 2015. "Results from the International Consensus Conference on Myo-inositol and d-chiro-inositol in Obstetrics and Gynecology: the link between metabolic syndrome and PCOS." *Eur J Obstet Gynecol Reprod Biol* 195:72-6.

Fruzzetti, F., D. Perini, M. Russo, F. Bucci, and A. Gadducci. 2017. "Comparison of two insulin sensitizers, metformin and myo-inositol, in women with polycystic ovary syndrome (PCOS)." *Gynecological Endocrinology* 33 (1):39-42. doi: 10.1080/09513590.2016.1236078.

Genazzani, A. D., C. Lanzoni, F. Ricchieri, and V. M. Jasonni. 2008. "Myo-inositol administration positively affects hyperinsulinemia and hormonal parameters in overweight patients with polycystic ovary syndrome." *Gynecol Endocrinol* 24 (3):139-44. doi: 10.1080/09513590801893232.

Genazzani, A. D., C. Battaglia, B. Malavasi, C. Strucchi, F. Tortolani, and O. Gamba. 2004. "Metformin administration modulates and restores luteinizing hormone spontaneous episodic secretion and ovarian function in nonobese patients with polycystic ovary syndrome." *Fertility and Sterility* 81 (1):114-119.

Genazzani, A. D., A. Prati, S. Santagni, F. Ricchieri, E. Chierchia, E. Rattighieri, A. Campedelli, T. Simoncini, and P. G. Artini. 2012. "Differential insulin response to myo-inositol administration in obese polycystic ovary syndrome patients." *Gynecological Endocrinology* 28 (12):969-973.

Gerli, S., M. Mignosa, and G. C. Di Renzo. 2003. "Effects of inositol on ovarian function and metabolic factors in women with PCOS: a randomized double blind placebo-controlled trial." *Eur Rev Med Pharmacol Sci* 7 (6):151-9.

Gerli, S., E. Papaleo, A. Ferrari, and G. C. Di Renzo. 2007. "Randomized, double blind placebo-controlled trial: effects of myo-inositol on ovarian function and metabolic factors in women with PCOS." *Eur Rev Med Pharmacol Sci* 11 (5):347-54.

Homburg, R. 1996. "Polycystic ovary syndrome—from gynaecological curiosity to multisystem endocrinopathy." *Human Reproduction* 11 (1):29-39.

Hooper, N. M. 1997. "Glycosyl-phosphatidylinositol anchored membrane enzymes." *Clinica Chimica Acta* 266 (1):3-12.

Iuorno, M. J., D. J. Jakubowicz, J. P. Baillargeon, P. Dillon, R. D. Gunn, G. Allan, and J. E. Nestler. 2002. "Effects of d-chiro-inositol in lean women with the polycystic ovary syndrome." *Endocr Pract* 8 (6):417-23. doi: 10.4158/ep.8.6.417.

Karimzadeh, M. A., and M. Javedani. 2010. "An assessment of lifestyle modification versus medical treatment with clomiphene citrate, metformin, and clomiphene citrate–metformin in patients with polycystic ovary syndrome." *Fertility and Sterility* 94 (1):216-220.

Kennington, A. S., C. R. Hill, J. Craig, C. Bogardus, I. Raz, H. K. Ortmeyer, B. C. Hansen, G. Romero, and J. Larner. 1990. "Low Urinary chiro-Inositol Excretion in Non-Insulin-Dependent Diabetes Mellitus." *New*

England Journal of Medicine 323 (6):373-378. doi: 10.1056/NEJM199008093230603.

Kim, C.- H., Kyung- Ah Han, Han- Jin Oh, Kevin Eng- Kiat Tan, Radhakrishna Sothiratnam, Askandar Tjokroprawiro, and Marcus Klein. 2012. "Safety, tolerability, and efficacy of metformin extended- release oral antidiabetic therapy in patients with type 2 diabetes: An observational trial in Asia." *Journal of Diabetes* 4 (4):395-406.

Kurzthaler, D., D. Hadziomerovic-Pekic, L. Wildt, and B. E. Seeber. 2014. "Metformin induces a prompt decrease in LH-stimulated testosterone response in women with PCOS independent of its insulin-sensitizing effects." *Reproductive Biology and Endocrinology* 12 (1):98.

Legro, R. S., S. A. Arslanian, D. A. Ehrmann, K. M. Hoeger, M. H. Murad, R. Pasquali, and C. K. Welt. 2013. "Diagnosis and treatment of polycystic ovary syndrome: an Endocrine Society clinical practice guideline." *The Journal of Clinical Endocrinology & Metabolism* 98 (12):4565-4592.

Legro, R. S., R. J. Zaino, L. M. Demers, A. R. Kunselman, C. L. Gnatuk, N. I. Williams, and William C. Dodson. 2007. "The effects of metformin and rosiglitazone, alone and in combination, on the ovary and endometrium in polycystic ovary syndrome." *American Journal of Obstetrics and Gynecology* 196 (4):402-e1.

Li, Y., S. Xu, M. M. Mihaylova, B. Zheng, X. Hou, B. Jiang, O. Park, Z. Luo, E. Lefai, and J. Y. J. Shyy. 2011. "AMPK phosphorylates and inhibits SREBP activity to attenuate hepatic steatosis and atherosclerosis in diet-induced insulin-resistant mice." *Cell Metabolism* 13 (4):376-388.

Macklon, N. S., and B. Fauser. 2003. "Mild stimulation in *in vitro* fertilization." *Annals of the New York Academy of Sciences* 997 (1):105-111.

McGarry, J. Denis, and N. F. Brown. 1997. "The mitochondrial carnitine palmitoyltransferase system—from concept to molecular analysis." *European Journal of Biochemistry* 244 (1):1-14.

Morgante, G., R. Orvieto, A. Di Sabatino, M. C. Musacchio, and V. De Leo. 2011. "The role of inositol supplementation in patients with polycystic ovary syndrome, with insulin resistance, undergoing the low-dose gonadotropin ovulation induction regimen." *Fertil Steril* 95 (8):2642-4. doi: 10.1016/j.fertnstert.2011.01.035.

Naderpoor, N., S. Shorakae, B. de Courten, M. L. Misso, L. J. Moran, and H. J. Teede. 2015. "Metformin and lifestyle modification in polycystic ovary syndrome: systematic review and meta-analysis." *Human Reproduction Update* 21 (5):560-574.

Nestler, J. E., D. J. Jakubowicz, P. Reamer, R. D. Gunn, and G. Allan. 1999. "Ovulatory and metabolic effects of D-chiro-inositol in the polycystic ovary syndrome." *N Engl J Med* 340 (17):1314-20. doi: 10.1056/nejm199904293401703.

Nestler, J. E., and V. Unfer. 2015. "Reflections on inositol(s) for PCOS therapy: steps toward success." *Gynecol Endocrinol* 31 (7):501-5. doi: 10.3109/09513590.2015.1054802.

Papaleo, E., V. Unfer, J. P. Baillargeon, L. De Santis, F. Fusi, C. Brigante, G. Marelli, I. Cino, A. Redaelli, and A. Ferrari. 2007. "Myo-inositol in patients with polycystic ovary syndrome: a novel method for ovulation induction." *Gynecol Endocrinol* 23 (12):700-3. doi: 10.1080/09513590701672405.

Papaleo, E., V. Unfer, J. P. Baillargeon, F. Fusi, F. Occhi, and L. De Santis. 2009. "Myo-inositol may improve oocyte quality in intracytoplasmic sperm injection cycles. A prospective, controlled, randomized trial." *Fertil Steril* 91 (5):1750-4. doi: 10.1016/j. fertnstert.2008.01.088.

Raffone, E., P. Rizzo, and V. Benedetto. 2010. "Insulin sensitiser agents alone and in co-treatment with r-FSH for ovulation induction in PCOS women." *Gynecol Endocrinol* 26 (4):275-80. doi: 10.3109/09513590903366996.

Reynolds, J. E. F. 1982. *Martindale: The Extra Pharmacopoeia*: London, UK; The Pharmaceutical Press.

Rizzo, P., E. Raffone, and V. Benedetto. 2010. "Effect of the treatment with myo-inositol plus folic acid plus melatonin in comparison with a treatment with myo-inositol plus folic acid on oocyte quality and pregnancy outcome in IVF cycles. A prospective, clinical trial." *Eur Rev Med Pharmacol Sci* 14 (6):555-61.

Rotterdam, ESHRE/ASRM-Sponsored PCOS Consensus Workshop Group. 2004. "Revised 2003 consensus on diagnostic criteria and long-term health risks related to polycystic ovary syndrome." *Fertil Steril* 81 (1):19-25.

Serhal, P. F., D. M. Ranieri, A. Kinis, S. Marchant, M. Davies, and I. M. Khadum. 1997. "Oocyte morphology predicts outcome of intracytoplasmic sperm injection." *Human Reproduction (Oxford, England)* 12 (6):1267-1270.

Shahebrahimi, K., N. Jalilian, N. Bazgir, and M. Rezaei. 2016. "Comparison clinical and metabolic effects of metformin and pioglitazone in polycystic ovary syndrome." *Indian Journal of Endocrinology and Metabolism* 20 (6):805.

Stabile, G., I. Borrielli, A. Carducci Artenisio, L. M. Bruno, S. Benvenga, L. Giunta, A. La Marca, A. Volpe, and A. Pizzo. 2014. "Effects of the insulin sensitizer pioglitazone on menstrual irregularity, insulin resistance and hyperandrogenism in young women with polycystic ovary syndrome." *Journal of Pediatric and Adolescent Gynecology* 27 (3):177-182.

Strugaru, A.-M., G. Botnariu, L. Agoroaei, I.-C. Grigoriu, and E. Butnaru. 2013. "Metformin induced lactic acidosis–particularities and course." *The Medical-Surgical Journal* 117 (4):1035-1042.

Sun, T. H., D. B. Heimark, T. Nguygen, J. L. Nadler, and J. Larner. 2002. "Both myo-inositol to chiro-inositol epimerase activities and chiro-inositol to myo-inositol ratios are decreased in tissues of GK type 2 diabetic rats compared to Wistar controls." *Biochem Biophys Res Commun* 293 (3):1092-8. doi: 10.1016/s0006-291x(02)00313-3.

Unfer, V., E. Raffone, P. Rizzo, and S. Buffo. 2011. "Effect of a supplementation with myo-inositol plus melatonin on oocyte quality in women who failed to conceive in previous *in vitro* fertilization cycles for poor oocyte quality: a prospective, longitudinal, cohort study." *Gynecol Endocrinol* 27 (11):857-61. doi: 10.3109/09513590.2011.564687.

Unfer, V., J. E. Nestler, Z. A. Kamenov, N. Prapas, and F. Facchinetti. 2016. "Effects of Inositol(s) in Women with PCOS: A Systematic Review of Randomized Controlled Trials." *International Journal of Endocrinology* 2016:12. doi: 10.1155/2016/1849162.

In: Inositols
Editor: Vittorio Unfer
ISBN: 978-1-53614-912-8

Chapter 8

INOSITOLS IN ASSISTED REPRODUCTIVE TECHNOLOGIES (ART)

Tony T. Chiu*[*], *PhD
IVF Centre (Hong Kong), Hong Kong SAR, China

ABSTRACT

Inositols are natural molecules having a C6 sugar alcohol that belongs to the vitamin B complex group. There are nine possible stereoisomeric forms of inositols while Myo-inositol (MI) is the major component widely distributed in human tissues and cells. Another essential stereoisomer, D-chiro-inositol (DCI), is produced from MI via epimerization of its C1 hydroxyl group. MI constitutes more than 99% of inositols content in many cell types while DCI make up the remaining part. Earlier studies have suggested that MI and its derivatives are important components of the structural phospholipids of the cell membranes and are precursors of the second messengers of many metabolic pathways. MI serves as a precursor for the synthesis of phosphoinositides that constitutes the phosphatidylinositol (PtdIns) signal transduction system shown to regulate diverse cellular functions including cell proliferations. We have previously shown that concentrations of MI and 17β-Estradiol in human follicular

[*] Corresponding Author's Email: tony.chiu@ivf.hk.

fluids are significantly higher in mature follicles containing good quality oocytes. We have further demonstrated that MI may enhance the rate of meiotic maturation and subsequent developmental potential of maturing oocytes through the triggering of premature calcium transients and, in turn, may accelerate the cell cycle protein synthesis. A recent study has suggested that higher rates of MI/DCI in follicular fluids are correlated with good quality blastocysts. Results of this study are in line with our earlier observations that mouse oocytes treated with MI were shown to have an increase in both implantation rate and post-implantation viability. Studies using MI for treating PCOS patients and male with semen factors have all shown to have a positive effect of MI in improving the oocytes and semen quality.

Keywords: myo-inositol, D-chiro-inositol, follicular fluid, oestradiol, intracellular calcium release, oocyte and semen quality

INTRODUCTION

Inositols (hexahydroxycyclohexanes) are natural molecules having a 6-carbon ring with a hydroxyl group attached to each carbon of the ring. There are nine possible stereoisomeric forms of inositols, related to the epimerization of the six hydroxyl groups. These compounds play a huge variety of physiological functions, with a key regulatory role in cell physiology as inositol phospholipids (Di Paolo and De Camilli 2006) and may be found in organisms belonging to all the Kingdoms of Life. They are very old molecules linked to the beginning of the biological evolution. Even, it was speculated that they played a role in contributing to the origin of life. In this case the synthesis of the ancestor molecule must have occurred prebiotically (Saiardi 2017). Anyway, Archaea used inositols very early and this can explain its involvement in a great array of functions that are the result of a differentiated evolution until the appearance of amoebozoans and metazoans around 1000 million years ago (Michell 2008).

MYO-INOSITOL AND D-CHIRO-INOSITOL IN PHYSIOLOGY

As mentioned previously, inositols are one of the primordial molecules of living beings and after a long evolutionary process now they play a multiplicity of functions in eukaryotes (Michell 2007). Myo-inositol (MI), among the above cited stereoisomeric forms, is by far the most important and widely distributed in nature.

Its name comes from a Greek word, meaning 'muscle', because it was isolated in the cardiac muscle by Scherer in 1850 and then characterized by Maquenne in 1887 (Maquenne 1887, Scherer 1850). Another essential stereoisomer is D-chiro-inositol (DCI), produced from MI through the epimerization of its C1 hydroxyl group. They may be found in free form, biologically active, as well as part of structural lipids or second messengers. Many studies done in the eighties, suggested that inositols play an important role in cell morphogenesis and cytogenesis, lipid synthesis, structure of cell membranes and cell growth (Berridge and Irvine 1989, Downes 1989). MI constitutes more than 99% of inositols content in many cell types whereas DCI is the remaining part. MI is involved in processes including glucose metabolism and the regulation of cell proliferation (Berridge and Irvine 1989, Downes 1989, Downes and Macphee 1990). Whereas the activation of glucose transporters and glucose utilization take place under the regulation of MI, glycogen synthesis is mainly controlled through DCI (Huang et al. 1993, Sun et al. 2002). On the other hand, in the ovary, MI regulates glucose uptake and FSH signaling, while DCI modulates insulin-induced androgen synthesis (Larner, Brautigan, and Thorner 2010, Nestler and Unfer 2015). A substantial variability may be detected in muscle, fat and liver regarding their concentration of MI and DCI, and this variability depends on the distinct functions played by the two stereoisomers in each tissue. MI and DCI levels are actively kept by means of the transformation of MI to DCI under the control of a NAD-NADH-dependent epimerase depending on the tissue necessities.

After the binding of insulin to its receptor, the glycosyl-phosphatidylinositol lipids located on the outer leaflet of the cell membrane are hydrolysed and released. They are two different inositolphosphoglycans

(IPG), having either MI or DCI (MI-IPG and DCI-IPG). Such compounds then enter the cells and influence the intracellular metabolism, with the activation of central enzymes involved in oxidative and non-oxidative metabolism of glucose (Larner 2002). Though there are some differences between MI and DCI activities, both stereoisomers, included in IPG, significantly decrease insulin resistance, favouring an appropriate glucose metabolism (Ortmeyer 1996).

INOSITOL IN FERTILITY

It is noteworthy that inositol was found to play a pivotal role, at physiological level, in female and male fertility and as a molecule very effective to solve the problems related to human infertility, that is a worldwide problem with a negative medical and psychosocial impact on couples in reproductive age (Fisher and Hammarberg 2012). Infertility is defined as the inability to conceive naturally after one year of regular unprotected intercourse. Normally a young couple has a 25% chance to get pregnancy after 1 month of unprotected intercourse, whereas 90% of the couples have a probability to reach this goal by 1 year. Only 5% of them conceive between one and a half year and two years. Both males and females contribute to about 50% of couple infertility. Ovulatory dysfunction and male factors are among the most common causes of infertility, which is a condition that can affect very negatively the couple's life, so it is important to improve their reproductive health issue. In this field MI can support, in a satisfying way, people looking for pregnancy.

MYO-INOSITOL AND D-CHIRO-INOSITOL IN OOCYTE DEVELOPMENT: PHYSIOLOGY AND THERAPY

Whereas the effects of DCI are limited to insulin signalling transduction, MI exerts other noteworthy activities that are essential to oocyte quality and maturation. MI is actively introduced into mammalian cells, and among them we have to highlight oocytes and preimplantation embryos. Studies carried out in animals and humans demonstrated that MI levels in follicular fluid (FF) are positively correlated with oocyte quality and pregnancy outcome. We have to keep in mind that FF is a metabolically active microenvironment where oocytes are hosted and grow; it plays a pivotal role in the processes of fertilization and embryogenesis. It was found in mammals that MI levels in the female reproductive tracts are considerably higher than in blood serum (Lewin et al. 1982). Such evidence prompts us to think that MI plays a pivotal effect on the fertility and reproduction processes.

It was seen that LH/FSH activity is actively modulated by MI and Phospholipase-C, by means of increased release of inositol-1,4,5-P3 (IP3) (Matsuda et al. 2009). We may assume that increased availability of MI-phosphate may intervene in the modulation of LH, since MI-phosphate is necessary in GnRH agonist-mediated LH inhibition (Janovick and Conn 1994).

In the early development of mouse, at least two different membrane protein transporters are activated to increase the MI uptake and incorporation into phosphoinositides, that gradually rise, going from the one-cell stage to the blastocyst stage (Kwon et al. 1992, Higgins and Kane 2003, Kane, Norris, and Harrison 1992). In the development of the zygote, oscillations in the concentration of Ca^{2+}, due to PLC-dependent InsP3 production, have key roles, from egg activation at fertilization (Ajduk et al. 2008) to blastomere divisions (Stachecki and Armant 1996).

Moreover, IP3 is involved in the regulation of intracellular Ca^{2+} release from mitochondria, and in oocytes this activity needs a specific receptor subtype (IP3-R1) (Goud et al. 1999). We remark that oocyte sensitivity to Ca^{2+} fluctuations is at its maximum namely when the final stages of oogenesis occur. Oocyte maturation in rat was proved to be generated by Ca^{2+} release following IP3 injection (Lowther et al. 2009).

We carried out a study aimed at investigating whether the MI levels in human serum are important for the processes involved in the nourishment of the embryo and consequently in its physiological development (Chiu and Tam 1992). The embryotrophic properties of human serum were tested by an in vitro model of post implantation mouse embryos, previously developed by us (Tam et al. 1987). The effect of MI on the embryotrophic activity of human serum was studied by supplementing the suboptimal serum samples that were unsupportive of embryo growth with extra MI. Serum obtained from patients having successful IVF pregnancies generally supported better development of post implantation mouse embryos and contained higher levels of MI, particularly if the serum sample was collected during the IVF treatment cycle. Serum samples obtained from patients with aborted pregnancies, though supporting mouse embryo development, contained significantly lower concentrations of MI. An improvement of the embryotrophic properties with exogenous supplement, containing this molecule, was achieved in some but not all of the suboptimal serum samples studied. Therefore, we showed that MI may be a serum trophic factor responsible for promoting in-vitro development of preimplantation embryos.

Other studies demonstrated that MI is incorporated into phosphoinositides and inositol phosphates in rabbit embryos (Fahy and Kane 1993) and can enhance bovine blastocyst development from in-vitro culture with medium supplemented with MI (Holm et al. 1999). Taken together, the results from these studies support the notion that MI serves as a precursor for the synthesis of phosphoinositides. This constitutes the phosphatidylinositol (PtdIns) signal transduction system known to be involved in the regulation of diverse cellular functions including cell proliferation (Berridge and Irvine 1989). The importance of PtdIns cycle activation in transducing information of various types across the plasma membrane has become more and more apparent between the eighties and the nineties (Downes 1989, Berridge 1993). It is activated in response to hormonal or other types of stimuli, and involves a receptor-dependent hydrolysis of an inositol lipid precursor to generate the inositol 1,4,5-trisphosphate [Ins(1,4,5)P3]. This is a second messenger that regulates many types of cellular processes by modulating the release of intracellular Ca^{2+} in a variety of cellular systems (Berridge 1993). Although much of these data derive from studies of somatic cells (Rhodes et al. 1983, Menè et al. 1993) available scientific evidence, already known from the nineties, sustains that such crucial events are also related to gamete development, including oocyte maturation, fertilization, and early embryonic development (Mehlmann and Kline 1994, Jones, Carroll, and Whittingham 1995, Stachecki and Armant 1996, Yoon et al. 2017).

In a study carried by us (Chiu et al. 2002) a significant difference between the concentration of MI in FF and serum ($P < 0.001$) was found. These findings are consistent with other studies suggesting that the concentrations of MI are not the same among different body fluids (Lewin, Szeinberg, and Lepkifker 1973). It has been proposed that cellular MI homeostasis can be achieved by contributions from synthesis de novo, inositol phosphate re-cycling and accumulation from the extra- cellular environment (Gani et al. 1993). We have not only demonstrated that MI is found in human FF, but that its concentration is significantly higher in FF containing good quality oocytes than FF containing poor quality oocytes ($P < 0.001$). Since MI is a precursor of the phosphoinositides, we postulated that MI in FF may undergo metabolism to the inositol phospholipids and ultimately to Ins(1,4,5)P3 during the maturation process of human oocytes. Cells require a constant replenishment with phosphoinositides but only contain a small pool of inositol phospholipids (Downes and Macphee 1990). Inositol transport in different tissues and cultured cell lines can occur either by a diffusion process, mainly at high MI concentrations, or by a specific active transport system, as was demonstrated using bovine preimplantation embryos from two-cell to early blastocyst stages (Khatami 1988, Hynes, Sreenan, and Kane 2000).

A complex system of inositol transporters was detected in bacteria, protozoa, fungi, plants and animals. Such transporters are essential and allow inositol uptake and its intracellular distribution. We can classify them into two groups on the base of their transport mechanisms, that are sodium ion coupled or proton coupled. The first one includes two transporters, called SMIT1 and SMIT2, whereas the second one is named HMIT (Schneider 2015). Na^+/inositol transporters were so far only identified in animals, while H^+/inositol symporters were found in all eukaryotic kingdoms. Human inositol transporters, the Na^+-coupled SMITs as well as the H^+-dependent HMIT, are of medical interest due to their role in numerous diseases (Schneider 2015). Relating to the tissue distribution, SMIT2 RNA had been detected in brain, kidney, heart, skeletal muscle, spleen, liver, placenta, lung, leukocytes, neurons (Coady et al. 2002), small intestine (Aouameur et al. 2007), and oocytes (Bourgeois, Coady, and Lapointe 2005).

For its part, SMIT1 RNA expression of was found in brain, heart, kidney, lung (Wright, Hirayama, and Loo 2007) and bone tissue (Dai et al. 2011). In turn, HMIT is predominantly expressed in the brain, and at lesser extent in the adipose tissue and kidney (Uldry et al. 2001), but also in oocytes (Bourgeois, Coady, and Lapointe 2005). Concerning MI uptake by oocytes, Pesty et al. for the first time have demonstrated this active process in maturing mouse oocytes since 1994 (Pesty et al. 1994).

These data suggest that MI in FF, Ins(1,4,5) P3 and its receptors may play an important role during oocyte maturation in humans. The higher concentrations of MI in FF containing good quality oocytes show that an active transport of MI is required to maintain MI homeostasis when phosphoinositide turnover is stimulated during the course of development of a healthy follicle. Since nuclear and cytoplasmic maturation occur independently during oocyte maturation, these processes need to proceed in a closely integrated manner to ensure developmental competence of the oocyte. Studies from in-vitro maturation (IVM) of human oocytes have shown that most of the matured oocytes derived from IVM are developmentally incompetent, possibly due to incomplete cytoplasmic maturation (Trounson et al. 1998, Mikkelsen and Lindenberg 2001). Such a poor IVM outcome can be related to the lack of a methodology for in-vitro assessment of cytoplasmic maturation (Rutherford 1998). Studies from hamster (Fujiwara et al. 1993), mouse (Mehlmann and Kline 1994), and human oocytes (Goud et al. 1999) have shown an increase in the sensitivity of inositol trisphosphate-induced Ca2+ release mechanism during the course of oocyte maturation. In our study, there was a positive correlation between the amount of MI in FF and both the cell number and the morphological score of the developed embryos. Since embryos were transferred on day two, whilst surplus ones were cryopreserved during the course of this study, data regarding the further embryo development cannot be obtained. Nevertheless, the present results are in line with other studies suggesting that MI is required to enhance the developmental competence of maturing oocytes.

In our study (Chiu et al. 2002), we have found that higher level of MI in FF is associated with larger follicles in terms of FF volume as well as the 17β-Estradiol concentration in FF. Serum concentration of 17β-Estradiol and follicle size are routinely used as conventional parameters for monitoring follicular development and oocyte maturity during ovulation induction and IVF treatment (Mikkelsen, Smith, and Lindenberg 2000). Furthermore, it has been shown that 17β-Estradiol can exert a direct nongenomic effect on maturing human oocytes via the induction of intracellular Ca^{2+} oscillations (Tesarik and Mendoza 1995). These findings, together with our results, further support our present hypothesis that MI may represent one of the maturational factors in FF responsible for the in-vitro growth of human oocytes. Perhaps, the content of MI in FF may represent a more appropriate physiological indicator than FF volume for monitoring the status of the developing follicles.

In another study carried by us (Chiu et al. 2003), it was demonstrated for the first time that MI exerts a positive effect on meiotic maturation and developmental competence of maturing mouse oocytes in the absence of exogenous gonadotrophins. demonstrating a dose-dependent effect of MI on the normal kinetics of germinal vesicle breakdown (GVBD) and a significant increase in the proportion of mouse oocytes that can progress to full meiotic maturation. The enhancing effects of MI on the kinetics of GVBD of mouse oocytes observed in this study were in line with the previous evidence on the role of Ins(1,4,5)P3 and its receptor in maturing mouse oocytes (Mehlmann, Mikoshiba, and Kline 1996). The observation on the dose effects of MI on maturing mouse oocytes allows us to postulate that the uptake of extracellular MI may reach a threshold value above which the inositol transporter may become fully saturated. Besides, higher osmolarity can be induced in the culture medium from higher concentrations of MI (i.e., >40 mmol/l) possibly related to the organic osmolyte nature of MI (Matskevitch et al. 1998) and this may have a toxic effect on maturing oocytes. Previous studies have suggested that Ca^{2+} signals may trigger meiotic resumption in mammalian oocytes (Lefèvre, Pesty, and Testart 1995). However, consistent and direct evidence indicating Ca^{2+} as an essential mediator of meiotic resumption in mammals remains uncertain. In this study, we found that the onset of GVBD in spontaneous maturation after the removal of dbcAMP was not accompanied by a noticeable change in intracellular Ca^{2+} concentration. This is consistent with the findings from Tombes et al. (Tombes et al. 1992) in which no detectable Ca^{2+} change was seen in oocytes during the initial stages of spontaneous meiotic maturation, using the same strain of mouse as used in this study. It is possible that intracellular Ca^{2+} oscillations seen in mouse oocytes undergoing spontaneous maturation are not causally related with GVBD. Moreover, all oocytes were initially treated with dbcAMP, in an attempt to synchronize the onset of spontaneous maturation of the GV oocytes prior to confocal microscopy. It has been shown that dbcAMP can disrupt the intracellular Ca^{2+} signals with a much longer inter-spike interval in pre-GVBD mouse oocytes (Lefèvre, Pesty, and Testart 1995). Such an effect may account both for our failure to detect an intracellular Ca^{2+} rise in control oocytes prior to GVBD, and for the atypical Ca^{2+} oscillations observed in the control and MI-treated GV oocytes. In any case, conflicting opinions still exist regarding the association between nuclear and ooplasmic intracellular Ca^{2+} signals and the induction of meiotic resumption (Lefèvre, Pesty, and Testart 1995, Mehlmann, Mikoshiba, and Kline 1996). These discrepancies between different observations may be related to a number of factors, which include: (i) whether oocytes are matured with or without the presence of surrounding cumulus cells; (ii) whether maturation is spontaneous, or hormone driven; (iii) the different animal strains or species used; and (iv) the type of oocyte maturation medium used in the study. Nevertheless, the present results demonstrate that the majority of GV oocytes, that display spontaneous Ca^{2+} oscillations in both the control and MI treated groups, are capable of undergoing the full process of GVBD. This is consistent with the current concept that intracellular Ca^{2+} transients are a phenomenon of meiotically competent mouse oocytes (Homa 1995). Further studies are required to investigate whether differences in the maturation rates of GV oocytes to metaphase II stage exist between those with intracellular Ca^{2+} transients accompanying GVBD and those that undergo GVBD alone, amongst both control and MI-treated GV oocytes. Interestingly, a recent report has demonstrated that calcium current activity and calcium stores are associated with the quality and developmental competence of maturing bovine oocytes (Boni, Cuomo, and Tosti 2002). In the present study, we observed that spontaneous intracellular Ca^{2+} transients were initiated in the nuclear region and then spread globally towards the cortical area in control GV oocytes undergoing maturation in-vitro. The treatment of GV oocytes with an optimal dose of MI can produce an extra intracellular Ca^{2+} rise which is followed by a similar pattern of spontaneous Ca^{2+} oscillations, as seen in the controls. Taken together, our observations suggest that the exogenous MI may not only enhance the basic phospholipid turnover or activate the phosphoinositide metabolism that takes place on the oocyte membrane (Homa 1991), but may induce a similar phenomenon in the nucleus and ultimately produce Ins(1,4,5)P3, which initiates intracellular Ca^{2+} release. Such a mechanism is supported by a previous study which demonstrated the presence of the type-1 Ins(1,4,5)P3 receptor in the nuclear membrane, and the detection of Ca^{2+} release from nuclear stores (Pesty, Avazeri, and Lefèvre 1998). Furthermore, the recent detection of cytoplasmic and nuclear phospholipase C-b1 and their relocation before the onset of GVBD have reinforced the notion that a nuclear phosphatidylinositol cycle may also be involved during resumption of meiosis in mouse oocytes (Avazeri et al. 2000). Our present observation on the small and scanty intracellular Ca^{2+} oscillations released in GV oocytes undergoing spontaneous maturation may be associated with the sub-optimal calcium release mechanism present in immature mouse oocytes (Carroll, Jones, and Whittingham 1996). Other studies have indicated that meiotically competent mouse oocytes develop an Ins(1,4,5)P3-induced Ca^{2+} release mechanism, possibly related to a structural reorganization of the endoplasmic reticulum, and with a concomitant increase in the number of cortical Ins(1,4,5)P3 receptors as they undergo the maturation (He et al. 1997, Mehlmann, Mikoshiba, and Kline 1996, Fissore et al. 1999). Indeed, different isoforms of Ins(1,4,5)P3 receptors have been detected in mouse oocyte, with the type I isoform being mainly associated with oocyte maturation (Parrington et al. 1998). Interestingly, when a monoclonal antibody against the Ins(1,4,5)P3 type I receptors is injected into the GV of the mouse oocytes, both the nuclear Ca^{2+} oscillations and GVBD are significantly suppressed, suggesting the presence of such receptors within the nuclei of these oocytes (Avazeri, Pesty, and Lefèvre 1998). Taken together, these findings provide further support for our postulation that MI may exert its enhancing effect on meiotic maturation via intracellular Ca^{2+} signals. Complete meiotic maturation of mammalian oocytes requires the proper intracellular changes associated with both the nuclear and cytoplasmic components of maturation. Although most of the morphological and biochemical changes during oocyte maturation are well documented, the identification of specific factors that bring about these changes is incomplete (Fulka, First, and Moor 1998). Maturation-promoting factor (MPF) has been well-documented to play a critical role in driving the oocyte meiotic cell cycle progression. Animal studies have shown that MPF is found in growing oocytes and its action seems to precede or coincide with GVBD (Homa 1995). In addition to MPF, mitogen-activated protein kinase (MAPK) has also been shown to participate in the regulation of cell cycle progression [Shimada, M., Zeng, W.X. and Terada, T. (2001) Inhibition of phosphatidylinositol 3-kinase or mitogen-activated protein kinase leads to suppression of p34cdc2 kinase activity and meiotic progression beyond the meiosis I stage in porcine oocyte surrounded by cumulus cells. Biol. Reprod., 65, 442-448]. However, the role of MAPK in meiotic resumption in mammalian oocytes remains to be determined (Shimada and Terada 2002). The fertilizability of the oocytes together with the acquisition of developmental capacity to 2-cell embryos, and preimplantation development are currently taken as an integral part of proper cytoplasmic maturation assessment. Fertilization failure seen in incompetent oocytes is often associated with successful sperm penetration but subsequent failure to from pronuclei. We have previously shown that some of the unfertilized human oocytes had cortical granules released after IVF (Tam, Loong, and Chiu 1990). Moreover, a recent study has provided the supporting evidence that unfertilized human oocytes have a high incidence of sperm penetration (Neuber and Powers 2000). The use of the Hoechst dye 33342 in this study has provided the evidence that a high proportion of non-activated oocytes are found amongst GV oocytes without exposure to MI during maturation. The inability of the in-vitro matured oocytes to become activated after sperm penetration may be related to incomplete cytoplasmic maturation of these oocytes (Fulka, First, and Moor 1998). In view of the potential occurrence of in-vitro 2-cell block in the majority of mouse strains (Muggleton-Harris, Whittingham, and Wilson 1982), and the fact that subtle imperfections during IVM can accurately be detected after implantation (Moor et al. 1998), the present study used our previously established model of post implantation embryo development (Tam et al. 1987) as the ultimate assessment of developmental competence and hence the quality of oocytes matured in vitro. Increasing evidence indicates that the type of culture medium and conditions of culture have a profound effect on the in-vitro development of preimplantation embryos (Ho et al. 1995, Niemann and Wrenzycki 2000). In fact, a recent study has revealed that in-vitro culture conditions can cause deviation from the normal mRNA expression pattern of the H19 gene in mouse embryos (Doherty et al. 2000). Because of the potential effects of culture conditions on embryonic development, the present study minimized the prolonged exposure of embryos to in-vitro culture conditions by transferring the embryos to the oviducts when they were at 2-cell stage. This can provide a more consistent and reliable test for the ultimate assessment of developmental competence of in-vitro matured oocytes. In this study, we showed that the proportion of fertilized oocytes with two pronuclei, the number of 2-cell embryos developed, and the percentage of normality of the post implantation embryos were significantly higher in GV oocytes cultured in maturation medium containing MI compared with control medium. To ensure that the effect of MI can only act on the maturation process of the oocytes, supplementation of MI is performed only in the maturation medium (MEM) but not in subsequent culture medium (M16). Thus, the improved outcome of meiotic maturation, fertilization, implantation and post implantation embryo development may reflect improvements in the quality of in-vitro matured oocytes due to MI exposure. Although the presumed effects of stimulation of PtdIns pathway on oocyte maturation remains to be elucidated, we have recently shown that higher concentrations of MI in follicular fluids are associated with good quality oocytes (Chiu et al. 2002). On the basis of our previous study and our present findings, we suggest that MI may well be enhancing the rate of meiotic maturation and subsequent development potential of maturing oocytes through triggering premature

Ca^{2+} transients that, in turn, may accelerate cell cycle protein synthesis and/or activity. Our present notion is further supported by the recent findings on the role of Ca^{2+}/calmodulin-dependent protein kinase II and Ca^{2+}-dependent protein kinase C in the regulation of meiotic resumption in mammalian oocytes (Downs, Cottom, and Hunzicker-Dunn 2001, Su and Eppig 2002). Further studies are warranted to investigate the association between the PtdIns pathway and levels of MPF and MAPK in order to provide a better picture of the enhancing effect of MI on mammalian oocyte maturation. It remains to be determined whether the generated Ca^{2+} signals can induce oocytes to reorganize the cytoplasmic environment in the second half of the meiotic maturation process, and this accounts for the oocyte's subsequent developmental capacity (Moor et al. 1998). In conclusion, the present study has demonstrated that the exposure of fully-grown mouse GV oocytes to MI during IVM can enhance meiotic maturation, and the subsequent developmental potential of these oocytes following fertilization. However, the differences in the proportion of normally implanted embryos found between oocytes matured in vitro (MI-treated) and in vivo suggest that factors other than MI are also required for optimizing the IVM system of mouse oocytes.

Furthermore, MI was shown to improve in vitro the quality and performance of embryo. Indeed, the inclusion of MI in human embryo culture media has recently been shown to increases the ability of in vitro produced and cultured mouse embryos to complete preimplantation development (Colazingari et al. 2014). Compared to embryos cultured in standard medium, embryos maintained in the presence of MI displayed a faster cleavage and developmental rate, leading to hypothesize the use of this molecule for human embryo culture in IVF cycles (Colazingari et al. 2014). A recent study (Ravanos et al. 2017) has related the concentrations of MI and DCI in FF to the quality of blastocysts. In this study the oocytes were taken from strictly healthy young women (egg donors, homogeneous for age and BMI, involved in a donation program), subjected to ovarian stimulation, whereas the sperm for fertilization was given by the male partner of each couple undergoing IVF (noteworthy, also recipients were homogeneous for age and BMI, and all the men were normospermic). FF specimens were allocated into two groups, correlated with grade 4+3 and grade 2+1 blastocysts, respectively. Data analysis allowed to define the good quality threshold related to the ratio between MI and DCI in FF as basically very close or higher than 70:1 (up to 100:1). The reduction of the ratio under this value was shown to exert negative consequences on blastocyst quality, assessed as grade 2 and 1. In summary, the authors found that good quality blastocysts, as shown by the grade assigned (4 and 3), were correlated with higher rates of MI/DCI found in FF, with satisfying results in IVF, conversely, poor-quality blastocysts, i.e., with low grade (2 and 1), were associated with lower rates of MI/DCI found in FF and negative outcomes in IVF. The authors did not find correlations between FF volume (i.e., the follicular volume) and its MI content, differently from our study [Chiu et al. 2002]. Their explanation was that such disagreement in the results might be due to the different physiologic features of the FF donors: in their study, enrolled subjects were fertile healthy women, aged 23.8 ± 3.2 years, whereas in our study two groups of women, aged 33.7 ± 3.5 and 33.8 ± 4.1 years (mean and SD) with fertility problems, were included. Overall, these data suggest that a higher MI/DCI ratio in FF correlates positively with good quality blastocysts, and the authors propose to consider them a promising parameter for the success of embryo implantation and pregnancy in ICSI.

These findings are very useful for PCOS patients looking for pregnancy. As well known, PCOS patients have several comorbidities, and one of them regards the IVF procedures. In fact, when they undergo ovarian stimulation, they are subjected to an increased risk of failure of the IVF cycle due to poor oocyte/embryo quality and/or increased risk of ovarian hyperstimulation syndrome (OHSS). The clinical trials so far performed show that MI pretreatment beginning three months before the onset of ovarian stimulation results in significant improvements in hormonal responses (Ciotta et al. 2011, Papaleo et al. 2009, Rizzo, Raffone, and Benedetto 2010, Unfer et al. 2011). In particular, MI reduces the amount of FSH necessary for optimal follicle development as well as serum levels of 17β-estradiol measured the day of hCG injection. This reduces the chance of OHSS also reducing the number of cancelled cycles. For these reasons, pretreatment of the patients with MI appears really promising. As for the biological outcomes of these trials, we have already indicated that MI treatment improves oocyte quality, by reducing, as shown by a growing number of trials, the number of degenerated and immature oocyte, in this way increasing the quality of embryos produced after fertilization of these cells (Ciotta et al. 2011, Papaleo et al. 2009, Rizzo, Raffone, and Benedetto 2010, Unfer et al. 2011). The effect of MI has also been tested in women not affected by PCOS but undergoing fertility treatment due to male factor or tubal factor. Beneficial effects highlighted in the treatment of PCOS women have also been confirmed in this setting, with particular reference to reduced amounts of FSH administered in order to obtain proper ovarian stimulation, furthermore, a promising trend in increasing clinical pregnancy has been highlighted (Lisi et al. 2012). Noteworthy, this result, confirmed in both PCOS patients and non-PCOS women, resembles our observation (Chiu et al. 2002), demonstrating that the amount of gonadotropin used for ovarian stimulation is reduced in women whose FF contains higher amounts of MI.

Inositol therapy was demonstrated a safe and effective therapy for enhancing oocyte follicular development and oocyte maturation and in stimulation and pregnancy outcomes in IVF procedures, and it was shown also in PCOS patients, as proven by many studies [for a comprehensive review see: (Unfer et al. 2016)].

MYO-INOSITOL IN SPERM DEVELOPMENT AND ACTIVITY: PHYSIOLOGY AND THERAPY

In male infertility, besides conditions such as varicocele, cryptorchidism, and hypogonadism, a significant proportion of infertility is undiagnosed, and it is mentioned as idiopathic infertility, characterized by sperm parameters below the World Health Organization (WHO) reference values (Organization 2010): i.e., oligozoospermia, asthenozoospermia and/or teratozoospermia (OAT). Idiopathic infertility affects between 25-30% of infertile patients (Quaas and Dokras 2008). It is noteworthy that male infertility had a significant increase over the past decades (Kumar and Singh

2015). Among the molecular mechanisms underlying male infertility, the oxidative stress due to the overproduction of reactive oxygen species (ROS) and reactive nitrogen species (RNS), play a substantial role, which includes a wide array of conditions. Obviously, an improper lifestyle, such as alcohol abuse, drug addiction, smoking, leads to a reduced ability to fertilize. Also, environmental pollution (smog, radiation, industrial gasses) and a wrong nutritional behaviour (for instance an hyperlipidic diet, etc.) (Chitra et al. 2001, Latchoumycandane and Mathur 2002, Eskenazi et al. 2005, Singh and Jaiswal 2013). We have to highlight that spermatozoa are more susceptible than other cell types to the harmful effects of these molecules. In particular, ROS can affect motility, morphology and DNA stability. The role of ROS and RNS in the pathology of sperm activity was carefully studied in recent times. An important actor is nicotinamide adenine dinucleotide phosphate oxidase (NOX), situated in leukocytes or in spermatozoa, which produces superoxide then transformed to peroxide by dismutase. In fact, NOX is the most prolific font of ROS in sperm suspensions. Human spermatozoa are very sensitive to lipid peroxidation because their plasma membrane contains a great amount of polyunsaturated fatty acids; for this reason, hydrogen peroxide was found to be the most toxic oxidizing agent for human spermatozoa, though there are other causes that impair sperm function (Griveau and Le Lannou 1997). ROS can induce alterations in mitochondrial membranes, in such way compromising sperm function, since the damage of these organelles prevents the energy (ATP) production, essential for performing the function of spermatozoa (Armstrong et al. 1999). Mitochondrial membrane potential (MMP) and ROS levels are inversely connected, since ROS cause damage to the mitochondrial membrane and, conversely, the damaged mitochondrial membrane induces higher ROS production (Wang et al. 2003). Among the causes that favour the onset of damages during spermiogenesis as well as on mature sperms, we remind the peculiarity of these cells to have very low DNA repair mechanisms and small quantity of cytoplasmic antioxidant enzymes (most of them are lost in spermiogenesis). Furthermore, spermatozoa themselves produce ROS, and spend a long time as isolated cells (Agarwal, Makker, and Sharma 2008, Lewis and Aitken 2005, Chenoweth 2007, Prakash et al. 2014).

The sperm cells get the ability to move during the epididymal transit, and this process allow them to go from the vagina to the Fallopian tubes, so penetrating the cumulus oophorus and triggering all the processes of fertilization (Beauchamp, Galle, and Blasco 1984). Following the penetration into the cumulus oophorus of the ovum, the spermatozoon binds to the zona pellucida having intact its plasma membrane, after this step, the acrosome reaction occurs (Kopf and Gerton 1991), with the release of hydrolytic enzymes necessary to digest the zona pellucida. It permits the spermatozoon penetration into the oocyte with the subsequent fertilization (Breitbart and Spungin 1997). All these events are allowed by inositol that plays a central role in the process of penetration into oocyte and fertilization. It occurs by increasing the release of intracellular Ca^{2+} due to the protein kinase PKC activation (Roldan and Shi 2007).

As it was observed in female, MI levels in mammalian male reproductive tracts are higher in comparison to its concentrations in blood, with an increase starting from the caput toward the cauda epididymis (Eisenberg and Bolden 1964, Chauvin and Griswold 2004, Hinton, White, and Setchell 1980). In transgenic mice, low MI levels within epididymis was associated to reduced fertility (Yeung et al. 2013). In male sex organs FSH-responsive Sertoli cells are the main sources of MI which plays a key role in regulating motility, capacitation and acrosome reaction of sperm cells. Working on pathological sperm samples (e.g., those coming from OAT patients), it was found that MI absolutely needs to perform essential functions at extracellular and intracellular level. In fact, we know that sperm cells of OAT patients have low motility and higher levels of the enzyme inositol monophosphatase-1 (IMPA-1) (Cryns et al. 2008). Such enzyme induces the dephosphorylation of phosphatidylinositol (PI). An increased expression of IMPA-1 in asthenozoospermic patients can modify phosphatidyl inositol signalling pathway, inducing a reduction in sperm motility (Martinez-Heredia et al. 2008). The decreased cell mobility found in spermatozoa from oligoasthenoteratospermic patients is caused by "amorphous fibrous material" that totally covers them, and the treatment with MI was shown to reduce this amorphous material and the consequent semen viscosity (Colone et al. 2010). Also, the osmoregulation of seminal fluid is under MI control and some of the different osmotic patterns can significantly decrease sperm progressive motility and velocities (Liu, Clarke, and Baker 2006).

Besides the reduced motility, sperm cells of OAT patients are characterized by morphological abnormalities in mitochondria and the midpiece. MI treatment improved midpiece volume and reestablished mitochondrial cristae morphology, inducing a structural normalization of mitochondria (Colone et al. 2010). At the functional level, MI acts directly on mitochondria increasing the membrane potential (Condorelli et al. 2011). The MMP allows us to detect the presence of apoptosis in the cell, being a marker of programmed cell death, and it is undoubtedly related to sperm functional parameters (motility and so on) (Marchetti et al. 2004), as well as to the ability to fertilize the oocyte and embryo quality (Marchetti et al. 2012). For such reason can be used as fertility index. High values of MMP are related to the integrity of this structure and the optimal levels of activity, that means high cell viability. Confirming these morphological-functional data, treatment of sperm cells from both OAT patients and normal subjects with MI increases total and progressive motility, improving the recovery of cells usable in IVF cycles after swim-up (Condorelli et al. 2012). The usefulness of adding MI in vitro to sperm of patients with OAT can be seen also in its capability to increase the number of spermatozoa with high MMP, and to reduce the number of those having low MMP (Foskett 2010, Condorelli et al. 2011, Condorelli et al. 2012).

MI was found useful on fertility parameters not only in vitro, but also in vivo.

A double-blind, randomized, placebo-controlled trial was carried out to evaluate the efficacy and safety of MI and folic acid treatment by oral route in men affected by idiopathic infertility (Calogero et al. 2015). MI effects on sperm parameters and reproductive hormones were evaluated in men affected by idiopathic infertility at t 0 and 3 months of treatment. MI was able to restore serum gonadotropin and inhibin B levels to normal values and to increase sperm parameters in this kind of patients.

In a prospective longitudinal study (Montanino Oliva et al. 2016) carried out in asthenospermic males with metabolic syndrome (MS), patients were administered for three months with MI, L-carnitine, L-arginine and vitamin E, selenium, and folic acid. At the end of the treatment, MS as well as the hormonal and spermatic conditions, cause of male infertility, significantly improved. In another study, the same therapy was administered to male with reduced sperm motility (Dinkova, Martinov, and Konova 2017). A significant improvement in sperm motility was reported in 85.32% of the patients, and the average motility was enhanced from 20.31% (SD ± 8.5) to 27.98 (SD ± 9.69) by means of the treatment. Only 12.84% of the treated men have not got beneficial effect, whereas in 1.84% the motility worsened.

In another study, MI was added directly on sperm cells to test its effect on semen parameters of male patients undergoing *in vitro* fertilization (IVF) cycles (Gulino et al. 2016). MI treatment improved spermatozoa count and, most importantly for IVF cycle, spermatozoa count after density-gradient separation method both in normospermic patients and oligoasthenospermic patients. The best increase was found in oligoasthenospermic patients compared to normospermic patients; this result strongly sustains the role of MI therapy for the preparation of patients undergoing ART, by improving the outcome of semen parameters.

Noteworthy, in all the studies above quoted, no adverse effects were observed after MI treatment. To further support this aspect, we have to highlight that MI is listed as affirmed as Generally Recognized as Safe (GRAS) for human consumption by the U.S. Food and Drug Administration (FDA) under 21 CFR 184.1370, when used as a nutrient supplement, an ingredient for special dietary foods, or in infant formulas in accordance with good manufacturing practices.

CONCLUSION

In conclusion, these findings support the useful role played by inositol to improve the sperm mitochondrial function, with positive effects on sperm motility in patients with altered sperm parameters. Therefore, patients with idiopathic infertility could have a great advantage by MI. Obviously further researches are needed on the wide benefits due to MI supplementation for improving human fertility in ART.

REFERENCES

Agarwal, A., K. Makker, and R. Sharma. 2008. "Clinical relevance of oxidative stress in male factor infertility: an update." *Am J Reprod Immunol* 59 (1):2-11. doi: 10.1111/j.1600-0897.2007.00559.x.

Ajduk, Anna, Maria A. Ciemerych, Victoria Nixon, Karl Swann, and Marek Maleszewski. 2008. "Fertilization differently affects the levels of cyclin B1 and M-phase promoting factor activity in maturing and metaphase II mouse oocytes." *Reproduction* 136 (6):741-752.

Aouameur, Rym, Sandra Da Cal, Pierre Bissonnette, Michael J. Coady, and Jean-Yves Lapointe. 2007. "SMIT2 mediates all myo-inositol uptake in apical membranes of rat small intestine." *American Journal of Physiology-Gastrointestinal and Liver Physiology* 293 (6):G1300-G1307.

Armstrong, J. S., M. Rajasekaran, W. Chamulitrat, P. Gatti, W. J. Hellstrom, and S. C. Sikka. 1999. "Characterization of reactive oxygen species induced effects on human spermatozoa movement and energy metabolism." *Free Radic Biol Med* 26 (7-8):869-80.

Avazeri, Nathalie, Anne-Marie Courtot, Arlette Pesty, Clotilde Duquenne, and Brigitte Lefevre. 2000. "Cytoplasmic and nuclear phospholipase C-β1 relocation: role in resumption of meiosis in the mouse oocyte." *Molecular Biology of the Cell* 11 (12):4369-4380.

Avazeri, Nathalie, Arlette Pesty, and Brigitte Lefèvre. 1998. *The germinal vesicle of the mouse oocyte contains elements of the phosphoinositide cycle: What is their role at meiosis resumption?* Vol. 38.

Beauchamp, P. J., P. C. Galle, and L. Blasco. 1984. "Human sperm velocity and postinsemination cervical mucus test in the evaluation of the infertile couple." *Arch Androl* 13 (2-3):107-12.

Berridge, M. J., and R. F. Irvine. 1989. "Inositol phosphates and cell signalling." *Nature* 341 (6239):197-205. doi: 10.1038/341197a0.

Berridge, Michael J. 1993. "Inositol trisphosphate and calcium signalling." *Nature* 361 (6410):315.

Boni, Raffaele, Annunziata Cuomo, and Elisabetta Tosti. 2002. "Developmental potential in bovine oocytes is related to cumulus-oocyte complex grade, calcium current activity, and calcium stores." *Biology of Reproduction* 66 (3):836-842.

Bourgeois, Francis, Michael J. Coady, and Jean-Yves Lapointe. 2005. "Determination of transport stoichiometry for two cation-coupled myo-inositol cotransporters: SMIT2 and HMIT." *The Journal of Physiology* 563 (2):333-343.

Breitbart, H., and B. Spungin. 1997. "The biochemistry of the acrosome reaction." *Mol Hum Reprod* 3 (3):195-202.

Calogero, A. E., G. Gullo, S. La Vignera, R. A. Condorelli, and A. Vaiarelli. 2015. "Myoinositol improves sperm parameters and serum reproductive hormones in patients with idiopathic infertility: a prospective double-blind randomized placebo-controlled study." *Andrology* 3 (3):491-5. doi: 10.1111/andr.12025.

Carroll, John, Keith T. Jones, and David G. Whittingham. 1996. "Ca2+ release and the development of Ca2+ release mechanisms during oocyte maturation: a prelude to fertilization." *Reviews of Reproduction* 1 (3):137-143.

Chauvin, T. R., and M. D. Griswold. 2004. "Characterization of the expression and regulation of genes necessary for myo-inositol biosynthesis and transport in the seminiferous epithelium." *Biol Reprod* 70 (3):744-51. doi: 10.1095/biolreprod.103.022731.

Chenoweth, P. J. 2007. "Influence of the male on embryo quality." *Theriogenology* 68 (3):308-315. doi: https://doi.org/10.1016/j.theriogenology.2007.04.002.

Chitra, K. C., R. Sujatha, C. Latchoumycandane, and P. P. Mathur. 2001. "Effect of lindane on antioxidant enzymes in epididymis and epididymal sperm of adult rats." *Asian J Androl* 3 (3):205-8.

Chiu, T. T., M. S. Rogers, E. L. Law, C. M. Briton-Jones, L. P. Cheung, and C. J. Haines. 2002. "Follicular fluid and serum concentrations of myo-inositol in patients undergoing IVF: relationship with oocyte quality." *Hum Reprod* 17 (6):1591-6.

Chiu, T. T., and P. P. Tam. 1992. "A correlation of the outcome of clinical in vitro fertilization with the inositol content and embryotrophic properties of human serum." *J Assist Reprod Genet* 9 (6):524-30.

Chiu, Tony Tak Yu, Michael Scott Rogers, Christine Briton-Jones, and Christopher Haines. 2003. "Effects of myo-inositol on the in-vitro maturation and subsequent development of mouse oocytes." *Human Reproduction* 18 (2):408-416.

Ciotta, L., M. Stracquadanio, I. Pagano, A. Carbonaro, M. Palumbo, and F. Gulino. 2011. "Effects of myo-inositol supplementation on oocyte's quality in PCOS patients: a double blind trial." *Eur Rev Med Pharmacol Sci* 15 (5):509-14.

Coady, Michael J., Bernadette Wallendorff, Dominique G. Gagnon, and Jean-Yves Lapointe. 2002. "Identification of a novel Na+/myo-inositol cotransporter." *Journal of Biological Chemistry* 277 (38):35219-35224.

Colazingari, S., M. T. Fiorenza, G. Carlomagno, R. Najjar, and A. Bevilacqua. 2014. "Improvement of mouse embryo quality by myo-inositol supplementation of IVF media." *J Assist Reprod Genet* 31 (4):463-9. doi: 10.1007/s10815-014-0188-1.

Colone, M., G. Marelli, V. Unfer, G. Bozzuto, A. Molinari, and A. Stringaro. 2010. "Inositol activity in oligoasthenoteratospermia--an in vitro study." *Eur Rev Med Pharmacol Sci* 14 (10):891-6.

Condorelli, R. A., S. La Vignera, S. Bellanca, E. Vicari, and A. E. Calogero. 2012. "Myoinositol: does it improve sperm mitochondrial function and sperm motility?" *Urology* 79 (6):1290-5. doi: 10.1016/ j.urology.2012.03.005.

Condorelli, R. A., S. La Vignera, F. Di Bari, V. Unfer, and A. E. Calogero. 2011. "Effects of myoinositol on sperm mitochondrial function in-vitro." *Eur Rev Med Pharmacol Sci* 15 (2):129-34.

Cryns, K., A. Shamir, N. Van Acker, I. Levi, G. Daneels, I. Goris, J. A. Bouwknecht, L. Andries, S. Kass, G. Agam, H. Belmaker, Y. Bersudsky, T. Steckler, and D. Moechars. 2008. "IMPA1 is essential for embryonic development and lithium-like pilocarpine sensitivity." *Neuropsychopharmacology* 33 (3):674-84. doi: 10.1038/sj.npp.1301431.

Dai, Zhijie, Sookja K. Chung, Dengshun Miao, Kam S. Lau, Alfred W. H. Chan, and Annie W. C. Kung. 2011. "Sodium/myo-inositol cotransporter 1 and myo-inositol are essential for osteogenesis and bone formation." *Journal of Bone and Mineral Research* 26 (3):582-590.

Di Paolo, Gilbert, and Pietro De Camilli. 2006. "Phosphoinositides in cell regulation and membrane dynamics." *Nature* 443 (7112):651.

Dinkova, A., D. Martinov, and E. Konova. 2017. "Efficacy of myo-inositol in the clinical management of patients with asthenozoospermia." *Eur Rev Med Pharmacol Sci* 21 (2 Suppl):62-65.

Doherty, A. S., M. R. Mann, K. D. Tremblay, M. S. Bartolomei, and R. M. Schultz. 2000. "Differential effects of culture on imprinted H19 expression in the preimplantation mouse embryo." *Biol Reprod* 62 (6):1526-35.

Downes, C. P. 1989. *The cellular functions of myo-inositol*. Portland Press Limited.

Downes, C. Peter, and Colin H. Macphee. 1990. "Myo-Inositol metabolites as cellular signals." *European Journal of Biochemistry* 193 (1):1-18.

Downs, S. M., J. Cottom, and M. Hunzicker-Dunn. 2001. "Protein kinase C and meiotic regulation in isolated mouse oocytes." *Mol Reprod Dev* 58 (1):101-15. doi: 10.1002/1098-2795(200101)58:1<101::aid-mrd13>3.0.co;2-j.

Eisenberg, F., Jr., and A. H. Bolden. 1964. "Reproductive tract as site of synthesis and secretion of inositol in the male rat." *Nature* 202:599-600.

Eskenazi, B., S. A. Kidd, A. R. Marks, E. Sloter, G. Block, and A. J. Wyrobek. 2005. "Antioxidant intake is associated with semen quality in healthy men." *Hum Reprod* 20 (4):1006-12. doi: 10.1093/humrep/deh725.

Fahy, Mary M., and Michael T. Kane. 1993. "Incorporation of [3H] inositol into phosphoinositides and inositol phosphates by rabbit blastocysts." *Molecular Reproduction and Development* 34 (4):391-395.

Fisher, Jane R. W., and Karin Hammarberg. 2012. "Psychological and social aspects of infertility in men: an overview of the evidence and implications for psychologically informed clinical care and future research." *Asian Journal of Andrology* 14 (1):121.

Fissore, R. A., F. J. Longo, E. Anderson, J. B. Parys, and T. Ducibella. 1999. "Differential distribution of inositol trisphosphate receptor isoforms in mouse oocytes." *Biol Reprod* 60 (1):49-57.

Foskett, J. K. 2010. "Inositol trisphosphate receptor Ca2+ release channels in neurological diseases." *Pflugers Arch* 460 (2):481-94. doi: 10.1007/s00424-010-0826-0.

Fujiwara, Toshihiro, Ken Nakada, Hideki Shirakawa, and Shunichi Miyazaki. 1993. "Development of inositol trisphosphate-induced calcium release mechanism during maturation of hamster oocytes." *Developmental Biology* 156 (1):69-79.

Fulka, J., Jr., N. L. First, and R. M. Moor. 1998. "Nuclear and cytoplasmic determinants involved in the regulation of mammalian oocyte maturation." *Mol Hum Reprod* 4 (1):41-9.

Gani, David, C. Peter Downes, Ian Batty, and Janice Bramham. 1993. "Lithium and myo-inositol homeostasis." *Biochimica et Biophysica Acta (BBA)-Molecular Cell Research* 1177 (3):253-269.

Goud, Pravin T., Anuradha P. Goud, Patric Van Oostveldt, and Marc Dhont. 1999. "Presence and dynamic redistribution of type I inositol 1, 4, 5-trisphosphate receptors in human oocytes and embryos during in-vitro maturation, fertilization and early cleavage divisions." *Molecular Human Reproduction* 5 (5):441-451.

Griveau, J. F., and D. Le Lannou. 1997. "Reactive oxygen species and human spermatozoa: physiology and pathology." *Int J Androl* 20 (2): 61-9.

Gulino, F. A., E. Leonardi, I. Marilli, G. Musmeci, S. G. Vitale, V. Leanza, and M. A. Palumbo. 2016. "Effect of treatment with myo-inositol on semen parameters of patients undergoing an IVF cycle: in vivo study." *Gynecol Endocrinol* 32 (1):65-8. doi: 10.3109/09513590.2015.1080680.

He, C. L., P. Damiani, J. B. Parys, and R. A. Fissore. 1997. "Calcium, calcium release receptors, and meiotic resumption in bovine oocytes." *Biol Reprod* 57 (5):1245-55.

Higgins, B. D., and M. T. Kane. 2003. "Inositol transport in mouse oocytes and preimplantation embryos: effects of mouse strain, embryo stage, sodium and the hexose transport inhibitor, phloridzin." *Reproduction* 125 (1):111-118.

Hinton, B. T., R. W. White, and B. P. Setchell. 1980. "Concentrations of myo-inositol in the luminal fluid of the mammalian testis and epididymis." *J Reprod Fertil* 58 (2):395-9.

Ho, Y., K. Wigglesworth, J. J. Eppig, and R. M. Schultz. 1995. "Preimplantation development of mouse embryos in KSOM: augmentation by amino acids and analysis of gene expression." *Mol Reprod Dev* 41 (2):232-8. doi: 10.1002/mrd.1080410214.

Holm, P., P. J. Booth, M. H. Schmidt, T. Greve, and H. Callesen. 1999. "High bovine blastocyst development in a static in vitro production system using SOFaa medium supplemented with sodium citrate and myo-inositol with or without serum-proteins." *Theriogenology* 52 (4):683-700. doi: 10.1016/s0093-691x(99)00162-4.

Homa, Sheryl T. 1991. "Neomycin, an inhibitor of phosphoinositide hydrolysis, inhibits the resumption of bovine oocyte spontaneous meiotic maturation." *Journal of Experimental Zoology* 258 (1):95-103.

Homa, Sheryl T. 1995. "Calcium and meiotic maturation of the mammalian oocyte." *Molecular Reproduction and Development* 40 (1):122-134.

Huang, L. C., M. C. Fonteles, D. B. Houston, C. Zhang, and J. Larner. 1993. "Chiroinositol deficiency and insulin resistance. III. Acute glycogenic and hypoglycemic effects of two inositol phosphoglycan insulin mediators in normal and streptozotocin-diabetic rats in vivo." *Endocrinology* 132 (2):652-7. doi: 10.1210/endo.132.2.8425485.

Hynes, A. C., J. M. Sreenan, and M. T. Kane. 2000. "Uptake and incorporation of myo-inositol by bovine preimplantation embryos from two-cell to early blastocyst stages." *Molecular Reproduction and Development: Incorporating Gamete Research* 55 (3):265-269.

Janovick, J. A., and P. M. Conn. 1994. "Gonadotropin-releasing hormone (GnRH)-receptor coupling to inositol phosphate and prolactin production in GH3 cells stably transfected with rat GnRH receptor complementary deoxyribonucleic acid." *Endocrinology* 135 (5):2214-2219.

Jones, Keith T., John Carroll, and David G. Whittingham. 1995. "Ionomycin, thapsigargin, ryanodine, and sperm induced Ca2+ release increase during meiotic maturation of mouse oocytes." *Journal of Biological Chemistry* 270 (12):6671-6677.

Kane, M. T., M. Norris, and R. A. Harrison. 1992. "Uptake and incorporation of inositol by preimplantation mouse embryos." *J Reprod Fertil* 96 (2):617-25.

Khatami, Mahin. 1988. "Carrier-dependent and carrier-independent uptake of myo-inositol in cultured retinal pigment epithelial cells: Activation by heat and concentration." *Biochemistry and Cell Biology* 66 (9):942-950.

Kopf, G. S., and G. L. Gerton. 1991. The mammalian sperm acrosome and the acrosome reaction. In: *Elements of Mammalian Fertilization*

Kumar, N., and A. K. Singh. 2015. "Trends of male factor infertility, an important cause of infertility: A review of literature." *J Hum Reprod Sci* 8 (4):191-6. doi: 10.4103/0974-1208.170370.

Kwon, H. Moo, Atsushi Yamauchi, Shinichi Uchida, A. S. Preston, A. Garcia-Perez, M. B. Burg, and J. S. Handler. 1992. "Cloning of the cDNa for a Na+/myo-inositol cotransporter, a hypertonicity stress protein." *Journal of Biological Chemistry* 267 (9):6297-6301.

Larner, J. 2002. "D-chiro-inositol--its functional role in insulin action and its deficit in insulin resistance." *Int J Exp Diabetes Res* 3 (1):47-60.

Larner, Joseph, David L. Brautigan, and Michael O. Thorner. 2010. "D-chiro-inositol glycans in insulin signaling and insulin resistance." *Molecular Medicine* 16 (11-12):543.

Latchoumycandane, C., and P. P. Mathur. 2002. "Induction of oxidative stress in the rat testis after short-term exposure to the organochlorine pesticide methoxychlor." *Arch Toxicol* 76 (12):692-8. doi: 10.1007/s00204-002-0388-9.

Lefèvre, Brigitte, Arlette Pesty, and Jacques Testart. 1995. "Cytoplasmic and nucleic calcium oscillations in immature mouse oocytes: evidence of wave polarization by confocal imaging." *Experimental Cell Research* 218 (1):166-173.

Lewin, Lawrence M., Arieh Szeinberg, and Elie Lepkifker. 1973. "Gas chromatographic measurement of myo-inositol in human blood, cerebrospinal fluid and seminal fluid." *Clinica Chimica Acta* 45 (4):361-368.

Lewin, Lawrence M., Ysca Yannai, Shlomo Melmed, and Mordechai Weiss. 1982. "Myo-inositol in the reproductive tract of the female rat." *The International Journal of Biochemistry* 14 (2):147-150.

Lewis, S. E., and R. J. Aitken. 2005. "DNA damage to spermatozoa has impacts on fertilization and pregnancy." *Cell Tissue Res* 322 (1):33-41. doi: 10.1007/s00441-005-1097-5.

Lisi, F., P. Carfagna, M. M. Oliva, R. Rago, R. Lisi, R. Poverini, C. Manna, E. Vaquero, D. Caserta, V. Raparelli, R. Marci, and M. Moscarini. 2012. "Pretreatment with myo-inositol in non polycystic ovary syndrome patients undergoing multiple follicular stimulation for IVF: a pilot study." *Reprod Biol Endocrinol* 10:52. doi: 10.1186/1477-7827-10-52.

Liu, D. Y., G. N. Clarke, and H. W. Baker. 2006. "Hyper-osmotic condition enhances protein tyrosine phosphorylation and zona pellucida binding capacity of human sperm." *Hum Reprod* 21 (3):745-52. doi: 10.1093/humrep/dei364.

Lowther, Katie M., Vanessa N. Weitzman, Donald Maier, and Lisa M. Mehlmann. 2009. "Maturation, fertilization, and the structure and function of the endoplasmic reticulum in cryopreserved mouse oocytes." *Biology of Reproduction* 81 (1):147-154.

Maquenne, Léon. 1887. "Sur les propriétés de l'inosite." *Comptes rendus hebdomadaires des séances de l'Académie des sciences* ["On the properties of inosite." *Weekly reports of sessions of the Academy of Sciences*] 104:297-299.

Marchetti, C., N. Jouy, B. Leroy-Martin, A. Defossez, P. Formstecher, and P. Marchetti. 2004. "Comparison of four fluorochromes for the detection of the inner mitochondrial membrane potential in human spermatozoa and their correlation with sperm motility." *Hum Reprod* 19 (10):2267-76. doi: 10.1093/humrep/deh416.

Marchetti, P., C. Ballot, N. Jouy, P. Thomas, and C. Marchetti. 2012. "Influence of mitochondrial membrane potential of spermatozoa on in vitro fertilisation outcome." *Andrologia* 44 (2):136-41. doi: 10.1111/j.1439-0272.2010.01117.x.

Martinez-Heredia, J., S. de Mateo, J. M. Vidal-Taboada, J. L. Ballesca, and R. Oliva. 2008. "Identification of proteomic differences in asthenozoospermic sperm samples." *Hum Reprod* 23 (4):783-91. doi: 10.1093/humrep/den024.

Matskevitch, J., C. A. Wagner, T. Risler, H. Moo Kwon, J. S. Handler, S. Waldegger, A. E. Busch, and F. Lang. 1998. "Effect of extracellular pH on the myo-inositol transporter SMIT expressed in Xenopus oocytes." *Pflügers Archiv* 436 (6):854-857.

Matsuda, Miho, Koushirou Tsutsumi, Takashi Kanematsu, Kiyoko Fukami, Yoshihiro Terada, Tadaomi Takenawa, Keiichi I. Nakayama, and Masato Hirata. 2009. "Involvement of Phospholipase C-Related Inactive Protein in the Mouse Reproductive System Through the Regulation of Gonadotropin Levels1." *Biology of Reproduction* 81 (4):681-689. doi: 10.1095/biolreprod.109.076760.

Mehlmann, Lisa M., and Douglas Kline. 1994. "Regulation of intracellular calcium in the mouse egg: calcium release in response to sperm or inositol trisphosphate is enhanced after meiotic maturation." *Biology of Reproduction* 51 (6):1088-1098.

Mehlmann, Lisa M., Katsuhiko Mikoshiba, and Douglas Kline. 1996. "Redistribution and increase in cortical inositol 1, 4, 5-trisphosphate receptors after meiotic maturation of the mouse oocyte." *Developmental Biology* 180 (2):489-498.

Menè, Paolo, Giuseppe Pugliese, Flavia Pricci, Umberto Di Mario, Giulio A. Cinotti, and Francesco Pugliese. 1993. "High glucose inhibits cytosolic calcium signaling in cultured rat mesangial cells." *Kidney International* 43 (3):585-591.

Michell, Robert H. *Evolution of the diverse biological roles of inositols.* 2007.

Michell, Robert H. 2008. "Inositol derivatives: evolution and functions." *Nature Reviews Molecular Cell Biology* 9 (2):151.

Mikkelsen, A. L., S. Smith, and S. Lindenberg. 2000. "Impact of oestradiol and inhibin A concentrations on pregnancy rate in in-vitro oocyte maturation." *Human Reproduction* 15 (8):1685-1690.

Mikkelsen, Anne Lis, and Svend Lindenberg. 2001. "Morphology of in-vitro matured oocytes: impact on fertility potential and embryo quality." *Human Reproduction* 16 (8):1714-1718.

Montanino Oliva, M., E. Minutolo, A. Lippa, P. Iaconianni, and A. Vaiarelli. 2016. "Effect of Myoinositol and Antioxidants on Sperm Quality in Men with Metabolic Syndrome." *Int J Endocrinol* 2016:1674950. doi: 10.1155/2016/1674950.

Moor, R. M., Y. Dai, C. Lee, and J. Fulka, Jr. 1998. "Oocyte maturation and embryonic failure." *Hum Reprod Update* 4 (3):223-36.

Muggleton-Harris, Audrey, D. G. Whittingham, and Lynette Wilson. 1982. "Cytoplasmic control of preimplantation development in vitro in the mouse." *Nature* 299:460. doi: 10.1038/299460a0.

Nestler, J. E., and V. Unfer. 2015. "Reflections on inositol(s) for PCOS therapy: steps toward success." *Gynecol Endocrinol* 31 (7):501-5. doi: 10.3109/09513590.2015.1054802.

Neuber, E., and R. D. Powers. 2000. "Is the mouse a clinically relevant model for human fertilization failures?" *Human Reproduction* 15 (1):171-174. doi: 10.1093/humrep/15.1.171.

Niemann, H., and C. Wrenzycki. 2000. "Alterations of expression of developmentally important genes in preimplantation bovine embryos by in vitro culture conditions: implications for subsequent development." *Theriogenology* 53 (1):21-34.

Organization, World Health. 2010. *Laboratory manual for the examination and processing of human semen*. Edited by 5. Vol. xiv. Switzerland: Geneva: World Health Organization, c2010.

Ortmeyer, Heidi K. 1996. "Dietary myoinositol results in lower urine glucose and in lower postprandial plasma glucose in obese insulin resistant rhesus monkeys." *Obesity Research* 4 (6):569-575.

Papaleo, E., V. Unfer, J. P. Baillargeon, F. Fusi, F. Occhi, and L. De Santis. 2009. "Myo-inositol may improve oocyte quality in intracytoplasmic sperm injection cycles. A prospective, controlled, randomized trial." *Fertil Steril* 91 (5):1750-4. doi: 10.1016/j.fertnstert.2008.01.088.

Parrington, J., S. Brind, H. De Smedt, R. Gangeswaran, F. A. Lai, R. Wojcikiewicz, and J. Carroll. 1998. "Expression of inositol 1,4,5-trisphosphate receptors in mouse oocytes and early embryos: the type I isoform is upregulated in oocytes and downregulated after fertilization." *Dev Biol* 203 (2):451-61.

Pesty, Arlette, Nathalie Avazeri, and Brigitte Lefèvre. 1998. "Nuclear calcium release by InsP3-receptor channels plays a role in meiosis reinitiation in the mouse oocyte." *Cell Calcium* 24 (4):239-251.

Pesty, Arlette, Brigitte Lefèvre, Jacek Kubiak, Gérard Géraud, Jan Tesarik, and Bernard Maro. 1994. "Mouse oocyte maturation is affected by lithium via the polyphosphoinositide metabolism and the microtubule network." *Molecular Reproduction and Development* 38 (2):187-199.

Prakash, Seppan, Elumalai Prithiviraj, Sekar Suresh, Nagella Venkata Lakshmi, Mohanraj Karthik Ganesh, Murugesan Anuradha, Lakshmanan Ganesh, and Premavathy Dinesh. 2014. "Morphological diversity of sperm: A mini review." *Iranian Journal of Reproductive Medicine* 12 (4):239-242.

Quaas, Alexander, and Anuja Dokras. 2008. "Diagnosis and Treatment of Unexplained Infertility." *Reviews in Obstetrics and Gynecology* 1 (2):69-76.

Ravanos, K., G. Monastra, T. Pavlidou, M. Goudakou, and N. Prapas. 2017. "Can high levels of D-chiro-inositol in follicular fluid exert detrimental effects on blastocyst quality?" *Eur Rev Med Pharmacol Sci* 21 (23):5491-5498. doi: 10.26355/eurrev_201712_13940.

Rhodes, D., V. Prpić, J. H. Exton, and P. F. Blackmore. 1983. "Stimulation of phosphatidylinositol 4, 5-bisphosphate hydrolysis in hepatocytes by vasopressin." *Journal of Biological Chemistry* 258 (5):2770-2773.

Rizzo, P., E. Raffone, and V. Benedetto. 2010. "Effect of the treatment with myo-inositol plus folic acid plus melatonin in comparison with a treatment with myo-inositol plus folic acid on oocyte quality and pregnancy outcome in IVF cycles. A prospective, clinical trial." *Eur Rev Med Pharmacol Sci* 14 (6):555-61.

Roldan, E. R., and Q. X. Shi. 2007. "Sperm phospholipases and acrosomal exocytosis." *Front Biosci* 12:89-104.

Rutherford, A. J. 1998. "The practical aspects of in vitro maturation of human oocytes." *Fertility and Reproductive Medicine*:577-587.

Saiardi, Adolfo. 2017. "Has Inositol Played Any Role in the Origin of Life?" *Life* 7 (2):24.

Scherer, Johann Joseph. 1850. "Uber eine neue aus dem Muskelfleisch gewonnene Zuckerart." ["About a new kind of muscle-derived sugar."] *Liebigs Annalen der Chemie* 73:322.

Schneider, Sabine. 2015. "Inositol transport proteins." *FEBS Letters* 589 (10):1049-1058. doi: https://doi.org/10.1016/j.febslet.2015.03.012.

Shimada, Masayuki, and Takato Terada. 2002. "Roles of cAMP in regulation of both MAP kinase and p34cdc2 kinase activity during meiotic progression, especially beyond the MI stage." *Molecular Reproduction and Development* 62 (1):124-131. doi: 10.1002/mrd.10075.

Singh, K., and D. Jaiswal. 2013. "One-carbon metabolism, spermatogenesis, and male infertility." *Reprod Sci* 20 (6):622-30. doi: 10.1177/1933719112459232.

Stachecki, James J., and D. Randall Armant. 1996. "Transient release of calcium from inositol 1, 4, 5-trisphosphate-specific stores regulates mouse preimplantation development." *Development* 122 (8):2485-2496.

Su, Y. Q., and J. J. Eppig. 2002. "Evidence that multifunctional calcium/calmodulin-dependent protein kinase II (CaM KII) participates in the meiotic maturation of mouse oocytes." *Mol Reprod Dev* 61 (4):560-9. doi: 10.1002/mrd.10034.

Sun, T. H., D. B. Heimark, T. Nguygen, J. L. Nadler, and J. Larner. 2002. "Both myo-inositol to chiro-inositol epimerase activities and chiro-inositol to myo-inositol ratios are decreased in tissues of GK type 2 diabetic rats compared to Wistar controls." *Biochem Biophys Res Commun* 293 (3):1092-8. doi: 10.1016/s0006-291x(02)00313-3.

Tam, P. P., E. P. Loong, and T. T. Chiu. 1990. "Localization of fucosyl glycoconjugates in human oocytes following insemination for in vitro fertilization." *J In Vitro Fert Embryo Transf* 7 (3):141-5.

Tam, Patrick P. L., Wood-yee Chan, Kenneth R. Mao, and Tony Chiu. 1987. "A correlative study on the embryotrophic property of patient's serum and the outcome of in vitro fertilization of human oocytes." *Fertility and Sterility* 48 (5):834-839.

Tesarik, J., and Carmen Mendoza. 1995. "Nongenomic effects of 17 beta-estradiol on maturing human oocytes: relationship to oocyte developmental potential." *The Journal of Clinical Endocrinology & Metabolism* 80 (4):1438-1443.

Tombes, Robert M., Calvin Simerly, Gary G. Borisy, and Gerald Schatten. 1992. "Meiosis, egg activation, and nuclear envelope breakdown are differentially reliant on Ca2+, whereas germinal vesicle breakdown is Ca2+ independent in the mouse oocyte." *The Journal of Cell Biology* 117 (4):799-811.

Trounson, A., C. Anderiesz, G. M. Jones, A. Kausche, N. Lolatgis, and C. Wood. 1998. "Oocyte maturation." *Human Reproduction* 13 (suppl_3):52-62.

Uldry, Marc, Mark Ibberson, Jean-Daniel Horisberger, Jean-Yves Chatton, Beat M. Riederer, and Bernard Thorens. 2001. "Identification of a mammalian H+-myo-inositol symporter expressed predominantly in the brain." *The EMBO Journal* 20 (16):4467-4477.

Unfer, V., J. E. Nestler, Z. A. Kamenov, N. Prapas, and F. Facchinetti. 2016. "Effects of Inositol(s) in Women with PCOS: A Systematic Review of Randomized Controlled Trials." *Int J Endocrinol* 2016:1849162. doi: 10.1155/2016/1849162.

Unfer, V., E. Raffone, P. Rizzo, and S. Buffo. 2011. "Effect of a supplementation with myo-inositol plus melatonin on oocyte quality in women who failed to conceive in previous in vitro fertilization cycles for poor oocyte quality: a prospective, longitudinal, cohort study." *Gynecol Endocrinol* 27 (11):857-61. doi: 10.3109/09513590.2011.564687.

Wang, X., R. K. Sharma, A. Gupta, V. George, A. J. Thomas, T. Falcone, and A. Agarwal. 2003. "Alterations in mitochondria membrane potential and oxidative stress in infertile men: a prospective observational study." *Fertil Steril* 80 Suppl 2:844-50.

Wright, E. M., B. A. Hirayama, and D. F. Loo. 2007. "Active sugar transport in health and disease." *Journal of Internal Medicine* 261 (1):32-43.

Yeung, Ching-Hei, Michael Anapolski, Iwan Setiawan, Florian Lang, and Trevor G. Cooper. 2013. "Effects of Putative Epididymal Osmolytes on Sperm Volume Regulation of Fertile and Infertile c-ros Transgenic Mice." *Journal of Andrology* 25 (2):216-223. doi: 10.1002/j.1939-4640.2004.tb02781.x.

Yoon, Jeong, Kyoung-Mi Juhn, San-Hyun Yoon, Yong Ko, and Jin-Ho Lim. 2017. "Effects of sperm insemination on the final meiotic maturation of mouse oocytes arrested at metaphase I after in vitro maturation." *Clinical and Experimental Reproductive Medicine* 44 (1):15-21.

In: Inositols
Editor: Vittorio Unfer
ISBN: 978-1-53614-912-8

Chapter 9

INOSITOLS AND PREECLAMPSIA

Marco Scioscia [*]
Department of Obstetrics and Gynaecology, Policlinico Hospital,
Abano Terme, Padua, Italy

ABSTRACT

Preeclampsia is a disease of human pregnancy characterized by hypertension and proteinuria. It may have a serious impact on pregnancy outcome, maternal health, and fetal wellbeing. Preeclampsia results from a complex interaction between immunological alterations, endothelial dysfunction, metabolic disturbances, and insulin resistance. Inositol derivates are known to be deeply involved in metabolic signaling and are highly expressed during preeclampsia on both maternal and fetal side. In the past two decades, several studies were published on different aspects where these molecules are involved and these studies demonstrated the relevance of inositols in many aspects of this syndrome. It appears that maternal increase of inositol phosphoglycans P-type in all tissues and fluids reflects an increased production of inositol mediators on the fetal side in preeclampsia that spill over the placenta into the maternal circulation contributing to the onset and mantainace of the syndrome.

[*] Corresponding Author's Email: marcoscioscia@gmail.com.

Keywords: inositol, preeclampsia, human pregnancy, metabolism, insulin messengers, eclampsia

INTRODUCTION

Preeclampsia is a reversible clinical phenotype characterized by pregnancy-induced hypertension and proteinuria and is a leading cause of maternal and perinatal morbidity and mortality in approximately 1 to 7% of pregnancies, with over 8 million cases worldwide per year (Steegers et al., 2010). Its incicence in high-risk pregnancies is as high as 25% and it is associated with a three and five fold increase of maternal and perinatal mortality risk, respectively. Despite much research, and clear improvement in our understanding of risk factors and pathogenetic mechanisms, the exact etiology of pre-eclampsia remains unknown. Preeclampsia is a severe complication of human pregnancy where immunology, metabolic alterations and systemic inflammation interact to determine hypertension, endothelial, and kidney damage. According to present knowledge, we can define preeclampsia as a non-linear disease as it is characterized by significant changes and multiple adaptations between the mother and the fetal/placental unit before and during overt clinical signs. Moreover, it is further complicated by preexisting factors such as genetic background, immunological diseases, metabolic alterations, and inflammatory diseases. In fact, the complexity of this disease appears evident in the heterogeneity of its onset, progression and clinical impact (Huppertz 2008; Redman and Sargent, 2010; Redman et al., 2014). The explanation of why the pathophysiology and, therefore, the cure of this severe complication of human pregnancy are still elusive. In the recent years, several papers focused on the exacerbated metabolic syndrome that occurs during preeclampsia and its role in augmented risks of cardiovascular and metabolic disease in later life (Steegers et al., 2010; Bokslag et al., 2016). Altered angiogenesis and increased insulin resistance seems to hold a pivotal role for long term complications (Wolf et al. 2004; Bokslag et al., 2016). This is supported by the observation that interventions to improve insulin sensitivity may reduce the risk of both hypertension in pregnancy and later life cardiovascular complications (Seely et al., 2003; Carpenter, 2007). It has been known since 2000 that some second messengers of insulin, namely inositol phosphoglycans (IPGs), were highly expressed during preeclampsia (Kunjara et al., 2000) and this has been proposed as a crucial link between endothelial dysfunction and insulin resistance in preeclampsia (Scioscia et al., 2015). Over these years, many studies on IPGs have been published and research has progressively moved from causative role to screening tests to endothelial dysfunction. Nevertheless, there remain several substantive concerns about this theory, upon which so much investigative effort has been based. This chapter on IPGs and preeclampsia with the support of other laboratory and clinical works may help to understand the present findings and to foresee future researches.

Inositol between Immunology and Metabolism

Inositol is involved in many cell functions, especially as a precursor of phophatidylinositol and phosphoinositides. Inositol second messenger system is deeply involved in metabolic and cell signaling pathways and mediates several insulin-like actions (Larner et al., 2010). Main signaling molecules of this family are present in eukaryotic cells as phosphoglycans incorporating myo- or D-chiro inositol (also known as IPG-A and IPG-P, respectively). They mediate different actions of insulin on glucose oxidative use and storage as IPG-A stimulates lipogenesis, activates acetyl-CoA carboxylase, inhibits cAMP-dependent protein kinase and modifies the activities of adenylate cyclase and cAMP-phosphodiesterase while IPG-P exerts specific insulin-mimetic properties on the glycogen metabolism through the activation of pyruvate dehydrogenase phosphatase, glycogen synthase phosphatase, and glycerol-3-phosphate acyltransferase (Varela-Nieto et al., 1996). IPG-P was supposed to have an important role in preeclampsia as it is highly expressed in all tissues (Scioscia et al., 2007) as summarized below. Apart from glucose metabolism (Gao et al., 2016), this molecule was shown to modulate insulin post-receptor signaling pathways involving IRS - PI3K - PKB/Akt (Insulin Receptor Substrate; Phosphatidyl Inositol 3-Kinase; Protein Kinase B) promoting trophic effects of insulin, enhancing protein synthesis, cell growth, differentiation, and cell survival (Lizcano and Alessi, 2002; Scioscia et al. 2014). These effects of inositols were demonstrated also in lymphocytes (Okkenhaug and Vanhaesebroeck, 2003; Huang and Sauer, 2010; Fayard et al. 2010; So and Fruman, 2012) where IL-2-inducible T cell kinase (ITK) and BTK (Bruton agammaglobulinemia tyrosine kinase) represent important mediators of PI3K signaling pathway respectively in T and B cells (Srivastava et al. 2013). PTEN and SHIP1 are two important phosphatase that dephosphorylate PtdIns(3,4,5)P3, the principal second messenger of PI3K, and their deficiency leads respectively to impaired T cell immune response and to severe myeloproliferative disorders and impaired NK cell function (Helgason et al., 1998; Suzuki et al., 2001; Suzuki et al., 2007; Suzuki et al., 2008). A fine balance between inositol phosphatases and PI3K is necessary for the proper activation and development of T cells (Srivastava et al. 2013). Uterine NK cells contribute to blastocyst implantation in species with invasive hemochorial placentation through secretion of cytokines, chemokines, and angiogenic factors prompting the physiological changes of the endometrium into decidual basalis and triggering cytotrophobalst invasion and spiral artery remodeling (Zhang et al., 2011). Jiang et al. (2000) reported that integrity of PI3K – MEK - ERK pathway is fundamental for degranulation in NK cells. This was confirmed by subsequent studies that demonstrated that inositol phospholipids have a prominent role in NK cell biology mainly through SHIP1 (Kerr and Colucci, 2011; Anderson et al., 2015). Apparently, PI3-K seems to run the critical phase in NK cells for antibody-dependent cellular cytotoxicity and for production of cytokines including IFNγ, TNFα, and granulocyte-macrophage colony-stimulating factor (GM-CSF) (Stahls and Carpen, 1989; Gumbleton and Kerr, 2013) as demonstrated in PI3-KR1-/- NK cells that resulted cytolytically incompetent (Awashi et al., 2008). Intracellular signaling in NK cells can be summarized as a sequence of phosphorylation/dephosphorylation of phosphatidylinositol (PI) that can trigger intracellular Ca2+ release (PI(4,5)P2 is hydrolyzed by phospholipase C into diacylglycerol to activate protein kinase C and inositol

1,4,5-trisphosphate), promote cytolytic competency, cytokine formation, chemotaxis, and modulate cellular metabolism (Gumbleton and Kerr, 2013). PKB/Akt modulates all these steps affecting the transcription and activity of phosphatase and tensin homolog (PTEN) that antagonizes PI3-K by converting PI-(3,4,5)P3 into PI-(4,5)P2 (Briercheck et al., 2015). The key role of PKB/Akt in NK cells was demonstrated indirectly by Kishimoto et al. (2007) in PTEN-deficient Vα14i NKT cells that resulted unable to produce IFNγ and to mount an effective response to cancer cells. Certainly, insulin-like growth factor 1 (IGF-1) that activates the classical postreceptorial IRS – PI3-K pathway play a role in the dynamic regulation and IFNγ production by maternal decidual NK cells (Hu et al., 2008).

INOSITOL PHOSPHOGLYCANS IN PREECLAMPSIA

Human pregnancy is characterized by a delicate equilibrium between physiological inflammation and insulin resistance as an adaptive response of the mother to the fetal/placental unit. A systemic inflammation secondary to placental oxidative stress is one of the most important maternal adaptations to fetus in early stages of pregnancy (Redman and Sargent, 2010). An alternative glucose metabolism has been proposed in human placenta in a low-oxygen environment in early pregnancy, mainly based on histiotrophic nutrition and non-oxidative catabolism of glucose (Burton et al., 2010). Inositol system has been proposed to hold a key role as a parallel signal pathway in this metabolic setting to promote insulin-like effects (glucose disposal and glycogen synthesis) to meet the needs of the fetus and the placenta (Burton et al. 2011). In preeclampsia a disruption of the equilibrium between an immune-mediated systemic inflammation, endothelial homeostasis and insulin resistance has been proposed (Redman and Sargent, 2003; Scioscia et al., 2015).

In this part of the paper we show the main findings on IPGs in all organs directly involved in preeclampsia in order to get a clear picture of the possible role of IPGs as a continuous adaptive response going from pre-gestational status to the development of preeclampsia. All the key organs involved in this complex disease like maternal liver (metabolism), endothelial and cardiovascular system, kidney (proteinuria), brain (eclampsia) on one side and fetus, placenta and amniotic fluid on the other side are closely knit in a single disease. Inositol second messengers in endothelial cells and cardiovascular system deserve a dedicated paragraph (below).

Since the beginning of pregnancy, an increase of IPG-P was demonstrated in healthy women compared to non-pregnant individuals (Scioscia et al., 2006) probably to meet metabolic needs as previously discussed. Urinary IPG-P levels continue to rise softly throughout pregnancy (as physiological insulin resistance does) with higher levels in clinically relevant insulin resistant states like gestational diabetes mellitus with a positive correlation with glycaemia (Scioscia et al., 2007). Urinary excretion of inositols was reported to be significantly increased in patients with chronic renal failure (Niwa et al., 1983). Notably, D-chiro inositol clearance was shown to exceed the creatinine clearance in insulin resistant subjects demonstrating an involvement of renal tubules besides the glomerulus (Ostlund et al., 1993; Tominaga et al., 2016). Proteinuria in pregnancy and preeclampsia is related to glomerular endotheliosis and proximal tubular defect and it is estimated that 40% or urinary proteins are glomerular in origin and 60% are tubular (Lindheimer and Kanter, 2010).

Preeclampsia shows an exacerbated insulin resistance secondary to excessive inflammation where increased maternal levels of IPG-P may represent a compensatory response to desensitization to insulin. In fact, pregnancy shows a physiological insulin resistant state associated with a raise of IPG-P urinary output under healthy conditions compared to non-pregnant women (Scioscia et al., 2006) and the excretion can augment in insulin resistant states (gestational diabetes mellitus and diabetes type 2) in parallel to maternal glycaemia (Scioscia et al., 2007; Scioscia et al. 2009). In a previous article of ours, we hypothesized that a physiological increase of IPG-P production during pregnancy allows a compensation to this "altered" metabolic state as demonstrated in non-pregnant subjects but when inflammation mounts during preeclampsia, the progressive increase of IPG-P production ends up "flooding" the intracellular signaling through the inactivation of some key molecules like IRS 1 and 2 (Scioscia et al., 2006). Interestingly, IPG-P was demonstrated to rise between 4 to 6 weeks before the onset of clinical symptoms (hypertension and proteinuria) reaching levels as high as 10 times higher than the physiological value (L'Omelette et al., 2018; Dawonauth et al., 2014; Paine et al., 2010; Williams et al., 2007). It is interesting to note that the longitudinal curve of IPG-P values in preeclamptic women is very similar to that reported for sFlt-1 by Levine et al. (2004). This may represent one of the key aspects of these molecules as they have the potential as a screening test and it throws an interesting light on the pathophysiology of the disease. In fact, if the raise of IPGs and sFlt-1 follow the pathophysiological changes that end up with hypertension and proteinuria (preeclampsia) then we may argue either that biochemical alterations develop over 4 to 6 weeks or first trimester events (shallow trophoblast invasion, primipaternity predisposition with altered immunological response at maternal/placental interface) were somehow tolerated in the first half of pregnancy and then the situation comes to a head later on. This may explain why we have not yet found any biomarker or sonographic finding as a reliable screening test in the first trimester (Huppertz, 2015). This hypothesis may apply also to sonographic findings in the first and second trimester that show that abnormal uterine artery Doppler can foresee the risk to develop early-onset preeclampsia but not the late-onset disease (Chien et al., 2000; Cnosse et al., 2008); we may argue that increased resistance in uterine arteries may be an expression of impaired vessel relaxation secondary to local acquired alterations (angiogenic, vasoactive and inositol mediators) more than structural anomalies of intrauterine arteries (modifications not exclusive to preeclampsia and found also in healthy pregnancy) and so foresee the development of the disease a few weeks later. According to this argumentation, all proposed markers of preeclampsia can identify women at risk only when processes that lead to maternal syndrome are started and develop over 4-8 weeks. Another and possibly more likely hypothesis is that different routes may lead to the development of preeclampsia.

Cerebral complications contribute substantially to mortality in preeclampsia (eclampsia, the most dangeours progression of preeclasia that presents with seizures and brain damage). Inositol phospholipid signaling in the maternal brain relies on extracellular uptake and recycling more than de novo synthesis as the key enzyme that converts glucose 6-phosphate to myo-inositol (MI) (that in turn can be epimerized to D-chiro inositol), namely myo-inositol-3-phosphate synthase (INO1), is confined to endothelial cells in brain vessels only (Wong et al., 1987) while inositol transporters (SMTIs and HMIT) are expressed in neurons of different brain regions (Di Daniel et al., 2006). Impaired autophagy was shown to contribute to epileptogenesis through the mechanistic (mammalian) target of rapamycin (mTOR), an enzyme belonging to the phosphatidyl inositol 3-kinase-related kinase family (Ghavami et al., 2014). Hyperactivation of this enzyme has been associated with temporal lobe epilepsy in humans and in animal models (Buckmaster et al., 2009; Zeng et al., 2009; Hartman et al., 2012; Sha et al., 2012; Macias et al., 2013). Altered concentrations of inositols was demonstrated to promote autophagy via mTOR-independent pathway and to increase Ca2+ release from the endoplasmic reticulum into the cytosol through inositol 1,4,5-trisphosphate receptor (Vicencio et al., 2009). Similar findings were reported in acute in seizure activity related to regulation of voltage-gated channel regulation (Viard et al., 2004), neuronal excitability (MacGregor et al., 2002), ion channels in synaptic plasma membranes (Lhuillier and Dryer, 2002), and epilepsy-related ion channel activity (Alberdi et al., 2015). Recently, MI was shown to be correlated with cerebral osmolytes in a proton magnetic resonance spectroscopy study (Nelander et al., 2018).

Placenta is fundamental for the pathogenesis of preeclampsia. Alterations of trophoblast invasion and spiral artery remodeling result from an altered immunological activity at the fetal-maternal interface. It has been hypothesized that abnormalities of the histiotrophic nutrition of trophoblast cells at early stages can be part of the process along with altered expression of vascular endothelial growth factor C (VEGF-C) by uterine NK cells (Burton et al., 2010; Robson et al., 2012). VEGF-C expression in uterine NK cells is regulated by PI3K/Akt signaling pathway (Zhang et al., 2012). During the first weeks of gestation, trophoblast invades endometrial glands and their lipid-rich secretions represent the first nutrients of human placenta (histiotrophic) before switching to hemotrophic nutrition (Burton et al., 2010). An alternative carbohydrate metabolism under low oxygen conditions was proposed and it involved inositol phosphoglycans mediators as a classical anaerobic glucose metabolism was not confirmed by studies on metabolites (Burton et al., 2011). Healthy human placenta was shown to contain more IPG-P than any other organ in non-pregnant subjects and the assessment of preeclamptic placental specimens gave a three-fold higher yields of IPG-P as measured through a specific bioassay procedure based on the activation of pyruvate dehydrogenase phosphatase (Kunjara et al., 2000). Placental vessels of mature intermediate villi from preeclamptic specimens were shown to be particularly enriched of this molecule especially in early onset preeclampsia compared to matched controls (Scioscia et al., 2012). Furthermore, the contemporary high concentration of IPG-P in the villous stroma in these samples suggested the hypothesis of an uptake of IPG-P from the fetus given the inability of placental tissues to produce these molecules (Deborde et al., 2003). Increased production of IPG-P in preeclampsia was proposed to be a compensatory mechanism for the increased maternal insulin resistance but actually it ends up impairing insulin signal transduction in the placenta when intracellular concentrations are very high as demonstrate in placental tissues by a serine phosphorylation of IRS (inactivation effect) (Scioscia et al., 2006). Probably the excessive accumulation of the mediator in placental tissue may induce an inhibitory effect flooding the insulin signal transduction itself. It is of some interest to note that although controversial results were reported in preventing preeclampsia with aspirin and statins, these medications were shown to prevent insulin receptor and IRS proteins from serine phosphorylation induced by different kinases (Gao et al., 2003; Lalli et al., 2008).

At that point, it seemed realistic that the increased IPG-P production during normal and preeclamptic pregnancy had the fetus as the main source. Studies on the fetal side revealed that amniotic fluid in healthy pregnancy contained a thousand times higher level of IPG-P than maternal urine (Scioscia et al., 2006) with a further increase during preeclampsia (Paine et al., 2006). Even fetal urine taken during the first trimester in non-preeclamptic women showed higher levels of IPG-P than maternal urine

(Scioscia et al., 2007). In active preeclampsia, the assessment of fetal serum confirmed that the circulating IPG-P was higher than in matched controls and this coupled with the evidence that infants of preeclamptic mothers had increased urinary excretion of the inositol mediator on the day of delivery (Scioscia et al., 2012). Therefore, it was postulated that a lipid form of IPG-P (that detected by ELISA test) was transferred from the fetal/placental unit to maternal circulation via exosomes (Burton et al., 2011). This is favored by a more permissive placental plasma membrane that shows thinner glycocalyx and less tight junctions (Sukhikh et al., 2016; Lievano et al., 2006).

INOSITOLS AND ENDOTHELIAL DYSFUNCTION

Endothelial dysfunction and circulating angiogenic factors heavily contribute to the pathophysiology of preeclampsia (Mutter and Karumanchi, 2008). Endothelial dysfunction is characterized by down-regulation of endothelial nitric oxide synthase levels, altered VEGF expression, acute atherosis, endoplasmic reticulum stress, enhanced inflammation and oxidative stress. Acute atherosis is characterized by lipid deposition and lipid-filled foam cells in the wall of the spiral arteries resulting from a dysregulation of immune response, inflammatory cytokines and angiogenic factors and it promotes endovascular clothes (Staff et al., 2014; Baltajian et al., 2014). Nevertheless, these lesions are not exclusive of preeclampsia cases but they can be found also in healthy pregnancy. Three important aspects can link this process to IPGs: (i) Inositol precursors, namely glycosyl-phosphatidyl-inositol anchors, were shown to regulate leukocyte interactions (polarization, crawling and diapedesis) with the luminal side of the vascular wall (Richardson and Fernandez-Borja, 2015), a fundamental step to atherosis; (ii) IPGs regulate oxidative, non-oxidative and lipogenic routes of glucose metabolism through the activation of different enzymes possibly with a relevant role in endothelial cell metabolism (Kunjara et al., 2016); (iii) Intracellular signaling pathways of angiogenic factors and inositol mediators interact in eukaryotic cells (Scioscia et al., 2015). As regards the latter aspect, PKB/Akt represents the molecule where the two intracellular pathways converge (Scioscia et al., 2014; Scioscia et al., 2015). Certainly, this serine/threonine protein kinase along with MAP/ERK (mitogen-activated protein kinase/extracellular signal–regulated kinase) hold a pivotal role in the regulation of many endothelial functions like cell hypertrophy and survival, migration, tube formation and nitric oxide production (Shiojima and Walsh, 2002; Ramos, 2008). Parenti et al. (1998) demonstrate that inhibition of the VEGF/PKB/Akt/eNOS pathway prevents VEGF-driven nitric oxide release and induces vasoconstriction. *In vitro* studies showed that D-chiro and MI can induce respectively the phosphorylation of PKB/Akt and MAPK/ERK kinases directly in human umbilical vein endothelial cells (HUVEC) in the absence of insulin (D'Oria et al., 2017). Both inositols were shown to be more active on PKB/Akt than insulin in human endothelial cells *in vitro* and this may potentiate the reported crosstalk between PKB/Akt and MAPK/ERK signaling pathways *in vivo*. In fact, Nascimento et al. (2006) reported that D-chiro inositol can reduce elevated reactive oxygen species in endothelial cells, increase vascular relaxation and preserve nitric oxide signaling in animal models through direct superoxide scavenging and metabolic actions. Supplementation with MI and D-chiro-inositol (DCI) has been shown *in vitro* to counteract lipotoxicity-induced autophagy and palmitate autophagy and senescence in human cardiac progenitor cells activating survival kinases (Akt and p42/p44 MAPK) (D'Oria et al., 2015).

SUMMARY OF NEW FINDINGS AND FUTURE PERSPECTIVES

Taken together, these findings suggest that IPG-P levels raise initially in pregnancy to compensate the physiological maternal insulin resistance and when insulin sensibility decreases for the augmentation of the systemic inflammation that occurs during preeclampsia, inositol mediators are produced and released in larger amounts as an attempt to restore insulin sensitivity (adaptive response). Unfortunately, the excessive mediator can impair many intracellular pathways that contribute to the maternal syndrome (altered trophoblast invasion, abnormal immune adaptation, impaired insulin signal transduction, proneness to seizures, endothelial dysfunction, and possibly with later cardiovascular disorders as proposed by Conti et al., (2013). Urinary IPG-P and serum angiogenic factors have the potential of good screening tests for preeclampsia even if they result elevate "only" within one to two months of the clinical onset of the disease. In fact, a closer monitoring and early diagnosis may prevent poor fetal and maternal outcomes.

Preeclampsia is not a linear disease. If we start from this assumption, the explanation of why the pathophysiology and, therefore, the cure of this severe complication of human pregnancy are still elusive. The pathophysiology of preeclampsia is very complex and has been only partially elucidated. The possibility to link all the events involved in the development of preeclampsia may suggest new aspects and promote integrated studies. Future researches on inositols may focus on their role in cardiovascular risk in patients with previous preeclampsia to complete the picture.

Furthermore, a key role of inositols in preeclampsia may be its possible use as a screening test. Indeed, preeclampsia is an appropriate disease for a screening test as certainly it is an important disease, with a definitive therapy (delivery) and, at early stages, the possibility to intensify maternal and fetal surveillance and to administer anti-hypertensive treatment to the mother to delay delivery. In fact, when preeclampsia develops late in the second trimester or early in the third trimester, thus between 25 and 32 weeks of gestation, there is a significant probability that the occurrence of development of intrauterine growth restriction (impaired fetal growth) and/or uncontrolled hypertension may require a preterm delivery. Uncontrolled hypertension may induce abruptio placentae with certain poor outcome (need for blood transfusion, emergency delivery and sometimes hysterectomy, clotting problems, fetal death, neurological consequences for the survival fetus). Impaired fetal growth and pretermission represent the main causes of neonatal demise.

As far as the economic impact is concerned, the costs of managing women with preeclampsia are enormous. In fact, treatment costs include not only the costs of prenatal care (repeated laboratory tests, sonographic fetal surveillance, prolonged antenatal hospitalization and time lost from work because of recommendations for bedrest) and delivery (delivery visits to control hypertension, induction of labour, emergency caesarean section) but also expenses after delivery (neonatal hospitalization for those fetuses born before term and/or with intrauterine growth restriction, neonatal and maternal follow-up tests and visits).

The diagnostic potential of this molecule was demonstrated in a recent case-cohort study showing a significant difference in urinary release of the lipid form of P-IPG between preeclamptic and healthy pregnant women well before the onset of symptoms. Whether this molecule is directly associated with the pathogenesis of preeclampsia is yet to be proven. Most researchers are convinced that the identification of a valid predictive marker for preeclampsia should be based on the knowledge of mechanisms of the disease (Mignini et al., 2005). We are not convinced of this assumption. If we analyse the problem from different points of view, we can even argue that this assumption is wrong. At present, the cause of preeclampsia remains unresolved, despite countless efforts have been done over the past decades. The pathophysiologic abnormalities of this syndrome are so heterogeneous and variable that an inverse approach may be the most appropriate. If we know that endothelial dysfunction and insulin resistance represent definite aspects of this syndrome, the study of these manifestations may lead to the development of a valid screening test and, perhaps to identify the causes of this disorder of human pregnancy. Indeed, a complex network of relationships (immunological, vascular, metabolic, and genetic aspects) is involved in the pathogenesis of this multi-organ disorder and this represents the most challenging side of this disease.

Therefore, laboratory research should aim to devise a novel screening test using a new methodological approach to the problem. In the past decade, we focused our attention on insulin resistance and preeclampsia. We have been able to identify a molecule (P-IPG) that seemed to have great potential for the development of a screening test and to possibly help to unravel the aetiology of this disorder.

REFERENCES

Anderson, C. K., A. I. Salter, L. E. Toussaint, E. C. Reilly, C. Fugère, N. Srivastava, W. G. Kerr, and L. Brossay. 2015. "Role of SHIP1 in Invariant NKT Cell Development and Functions." *J Immunol.* 195 (5):2149-56.

Awasthi, A., A. Samarakoon, X. Dai, R. Wen, D. Wang, and S. Malarkannan. 2008. "Deletion of PI3K-p85alpha gene impairs lineage commitment, terminal maturation, cytokine generation and cytotoxicity of NK cells." *Genes Immun* 9 (6):522-35.

Baltajian, K., J. L. Hecht, J. B. Wenger, S. Salahuddin, S. Verlohren, F. H. Perschel, Z. K. Zsengeller, R. Thadhani, S. A. Karumanchi, and S. Rana. 2014. "Placental lesions of vascular insufficiency are associated with anti-angiogenic state in women with preeclampsia." *Hypertens Pregnancy.* 33 (4):427-39.

Bokslag, A., M. van Weissenbruch, B. W. Mol, and C. J. de Groot. 2016. "Preeclampsia; short and long-term consequences for mother and neonate." *Early Hum Dev.* 102:47-50.

Briercheck, E. L., R. Trotta, L. Chen, A. S. Hartlage, J. P. Cole, T. D. Cole, C. Mao, P. P. Banerjee, H. T. Hsu, E. M. Mace, D. Ciarlariello, B. L. Mundy-Bosse, I. Garcia-Cao, S. D. Scoville, L. Yu, R. Pilarski, W. E. 3rd Carson, G. Leone, P. P. Pandolfi, J. Yu, J. S. Orange, and M. A. Caligiuri. 2015. "PTEN is a negative regulator of NK cell cytolytic function." *J Immunol.* 194 (4):1832-40.

Burton, G. J., E. Jauniaux, and D. S. Charnock-Jones. 2010. "The influence of the intrauterine environment on human placental development." *Int J Dev Biol.* 54 (2-3):303-12.

Burton, G. J., M. Scioscia, and T. W. Rademacher. 2011. "Endometrial secretions: creating a stimulatory microenvironment within the human early placenta and implications for the aetiopathogenesis of preeclampsia." *J Reprod Immunol* 89 (2):118-25.

Carpenter, M. W. 2007. "Gestational diabetes, pregnancy hypertension, and late vascular disease." *Diabetes Care.* 30 (2): S246-50.

Chien, P. F., N. Arnott, A. Gordon, P. Owen, and K. S. Khan. 2000. "How useful is uterine artery Doppler flow velocimetry in the prediction of pre-eclampsia, intrauterine growth retardation and perinatal death? An overview." *BJOG* 107: 196-208.

Cnossen, J. S., R. K. Morris, G. ter Riet, B. W. Mol, J. A. van der Post, A. Coomarasamy, A. H. Zwinderman, S. C. Robson, P. J. Bindels, J. Kleijnen, and K. S. Khan. 2008. "Use of uterine artery Doppler ultrasonography to predict pre-eclampsia and intrauterine growth restriction: a systematic review and bivariable meta-analysis." *CMAJ* 178: 701-711.

Conti, E., L. Zezza, E. Ralli, D. Caserta, M. B. Musumeci, M. Moscarini, C. Autore, and M. Volpe. 2013. "Growth factors in preeclampsia: a vascular disease model. A failed vasodilation and angiogenic challenge from pregnancy onwards?" *Cytokine Growth Factor Rev.* 24 (5):411-25.

D'Oria, R., L. Laviola, F. Giorgino, V. Unfer, S. Bettocchi, M. Scioscia. 2017. "PKB/Akt and MAPK/ERK phosphorylation is highly induced by inositols: novel potential insights in endothelial dysfunction in preeclampsia." *Hypertens Pregnancy* 10:107-112.

Dawonauth, L., L. Rademacher, A. D. L'Omelette, S. Jankee, M. Y. Lee Kwai Yan, R. B. Jeeawoody, and T. W. Rademacher. 2014. "Urinary inositol phosphoglycan-P type: near patient test to detect preeclampsia prior to clinical onset of the disease. A study on 416 pregnant Mauritian women." *J Reprod Immunol.* 101-102: 148-52.

Deborde, S., J. N. Schofield, T. W. Rademacher. 2003. "Placental GPI-PLD is of maternal origin and its GPI substrate is absent from placentae of pregnancies associated with pre-eclampsia." *J Reprod Immunol.* 59 (2):277-94.

D'Oria, R., L. Laviola, A. Leonardini, M. A. Incalza, C. Caccioppoli, P. Nigro, M. Scioscia, A. Natalicchio, S. Perrini, and F. Giorgino. 2015.

"Myo-Inositol and DCI Prevent Palmitate-induced Autophagy and Senescence in Human Cardiac Progenitor Cells." *Diabetes* 64: A137

Fayard, E., G. Moncayo, B. A. Hemmings, and G. A. Hollander. 2010. "Phosphatidylinositol 3-kinase signaling in thymocytes: the need for stringent control." *Sci Signal* 3:re5.

Gao, Y. F., M. N. Zhang, T. X. Wang, T. C. Wu, R. D. Ai, and Z. S. Zhang. 2016. "Hypoglycemic effect of D-chiro-inositol in type 2 diabetes mellitus rats through the PI3K/Akt signaling pathway." *Mol Cell Endocrinol.* 433: 26-34.

Gao, Z., A. Zuberi, M. J. Quon, Z. Dong, and J. Ye. 2003. "Aspirin inhibits serine phosphorylation of insulin receptor substrate 1 in tumor necrosis factor-treated cells through targeting multiple serine kinases." *J Biol Chem.* 278 (27):24944-50.

Gumbleton, M., and W. G. Kerr. 2013. "Role of inositol phospholipid signaling in natural killer cell biology." *Front Immunol* 4:1-8.

Helgason, C. D., J. E. Damen, P. Rosten, R. Grewal, P. Sorensen, S. M. Chappel, A. Borowski, F. Jirik, G. Krystal, and R. K. Humphries. 1998. "Targeted disruption of SHIP leads to hemopoietic perturbations, lung pathology, and a shortened life span." *Genes Dev.* 12 (11):1610-20.

Hu, Y., R. Tan, C. D. MacCalman, G. Eastabrook, S. H. Park, J. P. Dutz, and P. von Dadelszen. 2008. "IFN-gamma-mediated extravillous trophoblast outgrowth inhibition in first trimester explant culture: a role for insulin-like growth factors." *Mol Hum Reprod.* 14 (5):281-9.

Huang, Y. H., and K. Sauer. 2010. "Lipid signaling in T-cell development and function." *Cold Spring Harb Perspect Biol.* 2: a002428.

Huppertz, B. 2015. "Maternal-fetal interactions, predictive markers for preeclampsia, and programming." *J Reprod Immunol.* 108:26-32.

Huppertz, B. 2008. "Placental origins of preeclampsia: challenging the current hypothesis." *Hypertension* 51 (4):970-5.

Jiang, K., B. Zhong, D. L. Gilvary, B. C. Corliss, E. Hong-Geller, S. Wei, and J. Y. Djeu. 2000. "Pivotal role of phosphoinositide-3 kinase in regulation of cytotoxicity in natural killer cells." *Nat Immunol.* 1 (5):419-25.

Kerr, W. G., and F. Colucci. 2011. "Inositol phospholipid signaling and the biology of natural killer cells." *J Innate Immun.* 3 (3):249-57.

Kishimoto, H., T. Ohteki, N. Yajima, K. Kawahara, M. Natsui, S. Kawarasaki, K. Hamada, Y. Horie, Y. Kubo, S. Arase, M. Taniguchi, B. Vanhaesebroeck, T. W. Mak, T. Nakano, S. Koyasu, T. Sasaki, and A. Suzuki. 2007. "The Pten/PI3K pathway governs the homeostasis of Valpha14iNKT cells." *Blood.* 109 (8): 3316-24.

Kunjara, S., A. L. Greenbaum, D. Y. Wang, H. N. Caro, P. McLean, C. W. Redman, and T. W. Rademacher. 2000. "Inositol phosphoglycans and signal transduction systems in pregnancy in preeclampsia and diabetes: evidence for a significant regulatory role in preeclampsia at placental and systemic levels." *Mol. Genet. Metab* 69: 144-158.

Kunjara, S., P. McLean, L. Rademacher, T. W. Rademacher, F. Fascilla, S. Bettocchi, and M. Scioscia. 2016. "Putative Key Role of Inositol Messengers in Endothelial Cells in Preeclampsia." *Int J Endocrinol.* 7695648.

Lalli, C. A., J. R. Pauli, P. O. Prada, D. E. Cintra, E. R. Ropelle, L. A. Velloso, and M. J. Saad. 2008. "Statin modulates insulin signaling and insulin resistance in liver and muscle of rats fed a high-fat diet." *Metabolism.* 57 (1):57-65.

Larner, J., D. L. Brautigan, and M. O. Thorner. 2010. "D-chiro-inositol glycans in insulin signaling and insulin resistance." *Mol Med.* 16:543-52.

Levine, R. J., S. E. Maynard, C. Qian, K. H. Lim, L. J. England, K. F. Yu, E. F. Schisterman, R. Thadhani, B. P. Sachs, F. H. Epstein, B. M. Sibai, V. P. Sukhatme, and S. A. Karumanchi. 2004. "Circulating angiogenic factors and the risk of preeclampsia." *N Engl J Med* 350(7):672-83.

Lievano, S., L. Alarcon, B. Chavez-Munguia, and L. Gonzalez-Mariscal. 2006. "Endothelia of term human placentae display diminished expression of tight junction proteins during preeclampsia." *Cell Tissue Res.* 324: 433–448.

Lindheimer, M. D., and D. Kanter. 2010. "Interpreting abnormal proteinuria in pregnancy: the need for a more pathophysiological approach." *Obstet Gynecol.* 115: 365-75.

Lizcano, J. M., and D. R. Alessi. 2002. "The insulin signalling pathway." *Curr Biol.* 12 (7): R236-8.

L'Omelette, A. D., L. Dawonauth, L. Rademacher, P. Y. Robillard, M. Scioscia, S. Jankee, M. Y. Lee Kwai Yan, J. B. Razgia, and T. W. Rademacher. 2018. "New insights into early and late onset subgroups of preeclampsia from longitudinal versus cross-sectional analysis of urinary inositol-phosphoglycan P-Type." *J Reprod Immunol.* 125: 64-71.

Mignini, L. E., P. M. Latthe, J. Villar, M. D. Kilby, G. Carroli, and K. S. Khan. 2005. "Mapping the theories of preeclampsia: the role of homocysteine." *Obstet Gynecol.* 105 (2): 411-25.

Mutter, W. P., and S. A. Karumanchi. 2008. "Molecular mechanisms of preeclampsia." *Microvasc Res.* 75 (1): 1-8.

Nascimento, N. R., L. M. Lessa, M. R. Kerntopf, C. M. Sousa, R. S. Alves, M. G. Queiroz, J. Price, D. B. Heimark, J. Larner, X. Du, M. Brownlee, A. Gow, C. Davis, and M. C. Fonteles. 2006. "Inositols prevent and reverse endothelial dysfunction in diabetic rat and rabbit vasculature metabolically and by scavenging superoxide." *Proc Natl Acad Sci U S A.* 103 (1):218-23.

Nelander, M., A. K. Wikström, J. Weis, L. Bergman, A. Larsson, I. Sundström-Poromaa, and J. Wikström. 2018. "Cerebral Osmolytes and Plasma Osmolality in Pregnancy and Preeclampsia: A Proton Magnetic Resonance Spectroscopy Study." *Am J Hypertens.* 31 (7):847-853.

Niwa, T., N. Yamamoto, K. Maeda, and K. Yamada. 1983. "Gas chromatographicmass spectrometric analysis of polyols in urine and serum of uremic patients. Identification of new deoxyalditols and inositol isomers." *J Chromatogr* 277: 25–39.

Okkenhaug, K., and B. Vanhaesebroeck. 2003. "PI3K in lymphocyte development, differentiation and activation." *Nat Rev Immunol* 3: 317–30.

Ostlund, R. E. Jr, J. B. McGill, I. Herskowitz, D. M. Kipnis, J. V. Santiago, and W. Sherman. 1993. "D-chiro-inositol metabolism in diabetes mellitus." *Proc Natl Acad Sci U S A* 90: 9988–9992.

Paine, M. A., M. Scioscia, K. A. Gumaa, C. H. Rodeck, and T. W. Rademacher. 2006. "P-type inositol phosphoglycans in serum and amniotic fluid in active pre-eclampsia." *J Reprod Immunol.* 69 (2):165-79.

Paine, M. A., M. Scioscia, P. J. Williams, K. Gumaa, C. H. Rodeck, and T. W. Rademacher. 2010. "Urinary inositol phosphoglycan P-type as a marker for prediction of preeclampsia and novel implications for the pathophysiology of this disorder." *Hypertens Pregnancy.* 29 (4):375-84.

Parenti, A., L. Morbidelli, X. L. Cui, J. G. Douglas, J. D. Hood, H. J. Granger, F. Ledda, and M. Ziche. 1998. "Nitric oxide is an upstream signal of vascular endothelial growth factor-induced extracellular signal-regulated kinase1/2 activation in postcapillary endothelium." *J Biol Chem.* 273 (7):4220-6.

Ramos, J. W. 2008. "The regulation of extracellular signal-regulated kinase (ERK) in mammalian cells." *Int J Biochem Cell Biol.* 40: 2707-19.

Redman, C. W., I. L. Sargent, and A. C. Staff. 2014. "IFPA Senior Award Lecture: making sense of pre-eclampsia - two placental causes of preeclampsia?" *Placenta.* 35 Suppl: S20-5.

Redman, C. W., and I. L. Sargent. 2010. "Immunology of pre-eclampsia." *Am. J. Reprod. Immunol.* 63: 534-543.

Redman, C. W., and I. L. Sargent. 2003. "Pre-eclampsia, the placenta and the maternal systemic inflammatory response--a review." *Placenta* 24 Suppl A: S21-7.

Richardson, D. D., and M. Fernandez-Borja. 2015. "Leukocyte adhesion and polarization: Role of glycosylphosphatidylinositol-anchored proteins." *Bioarchitecture.* 5(5-6): 61-9.

Salzer, L., K. Tenenbaum-Gavish, and M. Hod. 2015. "Metabolic disorder of pregnancy (understanding pathophysiology of diabetes and preeclampsia)." *Best Pract Res Clin Obstet Gynaecol.* 29 (3):328-38.

Scioscia, M., K. Gumaa, S. Kunjara, M. A. Paine, L. E. Selvaggi, C. H Rodeck, and T. W. Rademacher. 2006. "Insulin resistance in hum preeclamptic placenta is mediated by serine phosphorylation of insu receptor substrate-1 and -2." *J Clin Endocrinol Metab* 91 (2):709-1

Scioscia, M., K. Gumaa, L. E. Selvaggi, C. H. Rodeck, and T. W. Rademacher. 2009. "Increased inositol phosphoglycan P-type in the second trimester in pregnant women with type 2 and gestational diabetes mellitus." *J Perinat Med.* 37 (5): 469-71.

Scioscia, M., K. Gumaa, M. Whitten, L. E. Selvaggi, C. H. Rodeck, and T. W. Rademacher. 2007. "Inositol phosphoglycan P-type in healthy and preeclamptic pregnancies." *J. Reprod. Immunol.* 76: 85–90.

Scioscia, M., S. A. Karumanchi, D. Goldman-Wohl, and P. Y. Robillard. 2015. "Endothelial dysfunction and metabolic syndrome in preeclampsia: an alternative viewpoint." *J Reprod Immunol.* 108: 42-7.

Scioscia, M., S. Kunjara, K. Gumaa, P. McLean, C. H. Rodeck, and T. W. Rademacher. 2007. "Urinary excretion of inositol phosphoglycan P-type in gestational diabetes mellitus." *Diabet Med* 24 (11):1300-4.

Scioscia, M., M. Nigro, and M. Montagnani. 2014. "The putative metabolic role of D-chiro inositol phosphoglycan in human pregnancy and preeclampsia." *J Reprod Immunol.* 101-102: 140-7.

Scioscia, M., P. Y. Robillard, D. R. Hall, L. H. Rademacher, P. J. Williams, and T. W. Rademacher. 2012. "Inositol phosphoglycan P-type in infants of preeclamptic mothers." *J Matern Fetal Neonatal Med.* 25 (2):193-5.

Scioscia, M., M. Siwetz, C. Campana, and B. Huppertz. 2013. "Differences in d-chiro-inositol-phosphoglycan expression between first and third trimester human placenta." *Pregnancy Hypertens.* 3 (1):1-2.

Scioscia, M., M. Siwetz, F. Fascilla, and B. Huppertz. 2012. "Placental expression of D-chiro-inositol phosphoglycans in preeclampsia." *Placenta* 33 (10): 882-4.

Scioscia, M., A. Vimercati, L. E. Selvaggi, C. H. Rodeck, and T. W. Rademacher. 2006. "Inositol phosphoglycan putative insulin mediator in human amniotic fluid." *J Matern Fetal Neonatal Med.* 19 (1):9-12.

Seely, E. W., and C. G. Solomon. 2003. "Insulin resistance and its potential role in pregnancy-induced hypertension." *J Clin Endocrinol Metab.* 88 (6): 2393-8.

Shiojima, I., and K. Walsh. 2002. "Role of Akt signaling in vascular homeostasis and angiogenesis." *Circ. Res.* 90 (12): 1243-50.

So, L., and D. A. Fruman. 2012. "PI3K signalling in B- and Tlymphocytes: new developments and therapeutic advances." *Biochem J* 442: 465–81.

Srivastava, N., R. Sudan, and W. G. Kerr. 2013. "Role of inositol polyphosphatases and their targets in T cell biology." *Front Immunol.* 23 (4): 288.

Staff, A. C., G. M. Johnsen, R. Dechend, and C. W. Redman. 2014. "Preeclampsia and uteroplacental acute atherosis: immune and inflammatory factors." *J Reprod Immunol.* 101-102:120-6.

Ståhls, A. K., and O. Carpén. 1989. "Generation of inositol phosphates during triggering of cytotoxicity in human natural killer and lymphokine-activated killer cells." *Scand J Immunol.* 29 (2): 211-6.

Steegers, E. A., P. von Dadelszen, J. J. Duvekot, R. Pijnenborg. 2010. "Pre-eclampsia." *Lancet* 376 (9741): 631-44.

Sukhikh, G. T., M. M. Ziganshina, N. V. Nizyaeva, G. V. Kulikova, J. S. Volkova, E. L. Yarotskaya, N. E. Kan, A. I. Shchyogolev, and V. L. Tyutyunnik. 2016. "Differences of glycocalyx composition in the structural elements of placenta in preeclampsia." *Placenta.* 43: 69-76.

Suzuki, A., K. Hamada, T. Sasaki, T. W. Mak, and T. Nakano. 2007. "Role of PTEN/PI3K pathway in endothelial cells." *Biochem Soc Trans.* 35 (Pt 2): 172-6.

Suzuki, A., T. Nakano, T. W. Mak, and T. Sasaki. 2008. "Portrait of PTEN: messages from mutant mice." *Cancer Sci.* 99 (2):209-13.

Suzuki, A., M. T. Yamaguchi, T. Ohteki, T. Sasaki, T. Kaisho, Y. Kimura, R. Yoshida, A. Wakeham, T. Higuchi, M. Fukumoto, T. Tsubata, P. S. Ohashi, S. Koyasu, J. M. Penninger, T. Nakano, and T. W. Mak. 2001. "T cell-specific loss of Pten leads to defects in central and peripheral tolerance." *Immunity* 14 (5):523-34.

Tominaga, T., R. K. Dutta, D. Joladarashi, T. Doi, J. K. Reddy, and Y. S. Kanwar. 2016. "Transcriptional and Translational Modulation of myo-Inositol Oxygenase (Miox) by Fatty Acids: Implications in renal tubular injury induced in obesity and diabetes." *J Biol Chem.* 291 (3): 1348-67.

Varela-Nieto, I., Y. Leon, and H. N. Caro. 1996. "Cell signalling by inositol phosphoglycans from different species." *Comp Biochem. Physiol B Biochem. Mol. Biol.* 115: 223-241.

Williams, P. J., K. Gumaa, M. Scioscia, C. W. Redman, and T. W. Rademacher. 2007. "Inositol phosphoglycan P-type in preeclampsia: a novel marker?" *Hypertension.* 49(1):84-9.

Wolf, M., C. A. Hubel, C. Lam, M. Sampson, J. L. Ecker, R. B. Ness, A. Rajakumar, A. Daftary, A. S. Shakir, E. W. Seely, J. M. Roberts, V. P. Sukhatme, S. A. Karumanchi, and R. Thadhani. 2004. "Preeclampsia and future cardiovascular disease: potential role of altered angiogenesis and insulin resistance." *J Clin Endocrinol Metab.* 89 (12):6239-43.

Zhang, J., Z. Chen, G. N. Smith, and B. A. Croy. 2011. "Natural killer cell-triggered vascular transformation: maternal care before birth?" *Cell Mol Immunol.* 8 (1): 1-11.

In: Inositols
Editor: Vittorio Unfer
ISBN: 978-1-53614-912-8

Chapter 10

INOSITOLS AND FETAL PROGRAMMING

Daniela Menichini*, MD and Fabio Facchinetti, MD

Mother Infant Department,
Clinical and Experimental Medicine PhD Program,
University of Modena and Reggio Emilia, Modena, Italy

ABSTRACT

The "Barker hypothesis" postulates that a number of organ structures and associated functions undergo programming during embryonic and fetal life, which determines the set point of physiological and metabolic responses that carry into adulthood. Hence, any stimulus or insult at a critical period of embryonic and fetal development can result in developmental adaptations that produce permanent structural, physiological and metabolic changes, thereby predisposing an individual to cardiovascular, metabolic and endocrine disease in adult life.

Intrauterine environment can be, for instance, perturbed by maternal dismetabolisms that negatively affect fetal development, causing adverse lifelong effects on offspring's health.

Inositols (Myo-inositol, MI and D-chiro inositol, DCI) are insulin sensitizer compounds that can play an important role by improving

* Corresponding Author's Email: daniela.menichini91@gmail.com.

maternal health, thus reducing the adverse effect of the fetal programming in the offspring born to mother affected by metabolic disorders, as obesity and metabolic syndrome (MS). Inositols at the rate 40:1 (MI:DCI) have been demonstrated to prevent maternal weight gain in an obese pregnant mouse model and to reduce hypertension, leptin levels also to improve the glucose homeostasis in a pregnant murine model of MS.

This combination of MI/DCI administered during pregnancy to mice with obesity and MS also reduced the adverse effects on cardiovascular and metabolic profile in the offspring, interrupting the vicious circle of obesity and metabolic disorders in the adult life of the future generations.

Thus, those findings suggest a promising role of MI and DCI in pregnancy complicated by metabolic disorders, by improving cardiovascular, metabolic and glucose profile in the mother and reducing metabolic diseases in the adult life of the offspring exposed in utero to a perturbated enviroment.

Keywords: inositol, fetal programming, obesity, pregnancy

INTRODUCTION

Fetal developmental programing is defined as the exposure of developing tissues or organs to an adverse stimulus or insults during critical period of fetal development that can permanently reprogram normal physiological responses in such a way to give rise to disease later in life.

Fetal programming occurs during embryonic and fetal development, a critical period in which tissues and organs are created. Insufficient nutrition during this time results in permanent alterations to certain structural and physiological metabolic functions of the fetus.

Human and animal studies have highlighted the link between the perturbation occurring in early-life development and increase susceptibility to obesity and related metabolic and cardiovascular disorders in later life. In particular, altered maternal nutrition, including both undernutrition and maternal obesity, has been shown to lead to transmission of metabolic disorders in their offspring, which can also perpetuate among generations.

This association has been conceptualized by Barker and Osmond in 1986 as the "Developmental origins of health and diseases" (DOHaD) also known as "The Barker's hypothesis" (Barker 1990) which states that environmental factors impacting the fetus during critical periods of development can cause adverse lifelong effects on offspring health. The critical period coincides with the timing of rapid cell differentiation (Widdowson and McCance 1975). Essentially, programming refers to the process of sustaining or affecting a stimulus or impairment that occurs at a crucial point in its development (Lucas 1994). Rickets has long demonstrated that undernutrition in the critical early stages of life brings about a continuing change in structure (Barker 1998a). The body's "memory" of undernutrition during the early stages of development translates into a pathology that determines future diseases (Barker 1995). This idea is based on animal studies that demonstrate how undernutrition in utero can alter blood pressure, cholesterol metabolism, insulin response to glucose, and other metabolic, endocrine, and immune functions important to human diseases (Barker 1998b; Lucas 1994; Barker 1995, 1998a).

Furthermore, recent studies have demonstrated that fetal programming can be a transgenerational phenomenon, transmitting the effects to subsequent generations, even in the absence of continuous environmental stressors, thus perpetuating the cycle of obesity and metabolic disorders in future generation (Benyshek 2013).

While the Barker hypothesis explains the maternal effects on the fetus via the abnormal uterine environment, genetics also play a role. The long-term health of the offspring depends on a gene–environment interaction, as it is determined by both the intrauterine environment (influenced by the maternal genetic makeup) and the genetic makeup of the fetus/offspring, which in turn includes some of the same genes inherited from the mother. Therefore, a genetic trait that regulates vascular function in the mother may indirectly affect the fetus by influencing utero-placental perfusion, as well as directly contribute to the long-term health of the offspring if inherited by the fetus (Barker et al. 1989, 2000; Barker 1997). The contribution of the maternal and paternal genes as well as epigenetic changes influence the fetal phenotype. Thus, the maternal contribution to the development of disease in later life may be either through the transmission of genetic factors, or through the development of the offspring in an abnormal uterine environment which might be operational in pregnancy complicated by hypertension, preeclampsia, diabetes (Chiossi et al. 2016).

MECHANISMS OF FETAL PROGRAMMING

Changes in endometrial endocrine, nutritional and cardiovascular conditions affect the expression of the fetal genome so it can adapt during development (Figure 1). Within this framework, the fetal genome determines the intrauterine growth potential, but actual growth is primarily determined by environmental effects, such as fetal nutrition and the hormonal environment (Godfrey 2002). Fetal programming can affect individual gene expression at any stage, from changes in molecular biological functions, such as receptor cell density or sensitivity, to permanent hormonal changes or even alterations in metabolism or responses to physiological stressors (Cunningham and Cameron 2003).

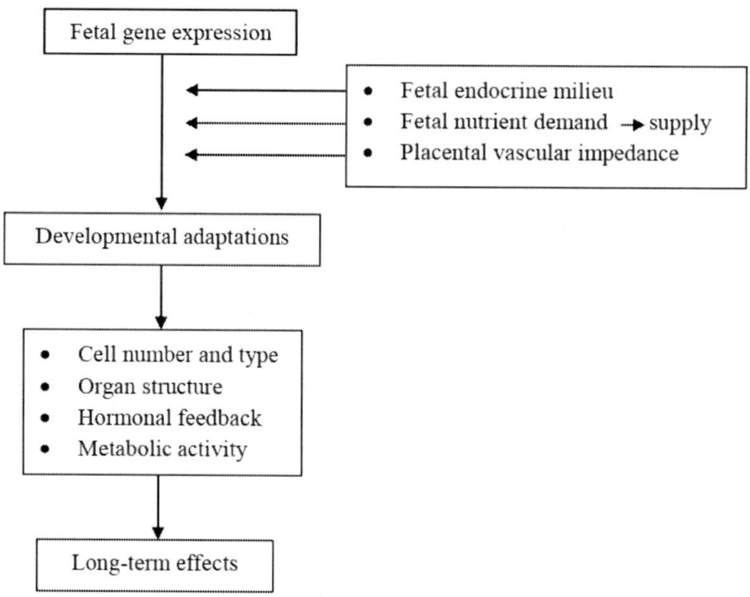

Figure 1. Fetal programming framework, indicating the possible role of the endocrine, nutrient, and cardiovascular milieu in utero.

There are several epigenetic mechanisms as:

- activation/inactivation of genes by DNA methylation, which suppresses gene expression;
- histone acetylation;
- chromatin remodeling regulatory feedback by microRNAs.

The perinatal acquired fetal and neonatal disorganization, due to the mis-programming, seems to be a consequence, at least in part, of elevated insulin levels during "critical periods" of pre- and early postnatal development. The metabolic, glycemic and hormonal regulatory factors, such as leptin, insulin, growth hormone, and growth factor, are epigenetically modulated and therefore, they significantly imprint the fetal programing, playing a crucial role in the development of diseases in adulthood. Thus, hormonal regulation and epigenetic mechanisms are complementary, acting as critical endogenous effectors that transmit environmental information to the genome, hormones, neurotransmitters and cytokines, as immune cell hormones, may play a decisive role in the processes of nutritional mis-programming.

New knowledge about these mechanisms involved suggests the development of new effective preventive and/or therapeutic options before and/or after birth. Thus, pregnancy and early infancy may provide an opportunity for intervention aimed at reducing later disease risk (Menichini, Longo, and Facchinetti 2018).

METABOLIC DISFUNCTIONS AND FETAL PROGRAMMING

MS and obesity are growing causes of morbidity and mortality worldwide. MS is a major risk factor for cardiovascular disease and is defined by the National Institutes of Health by having at least 3 of the following conditions: hypertension, elevated fasting plasma glucose, central obesity, elevated triglycerides, or low high-density lipoprotein cholesterol. MS etiopathogenesis and long-term consequences are still largely unknown, and preventive strategies have not yet been identified (Hutcheson and Rocic 2012). The impact of MS and obesity during pregnancy is substantial: indeed, all metabolic changes that develop during pregnancy have well-known effects on not only maternal and fetal health during pregnancy, but they also act as a catalyst for future health throughout later life (Catalano and Ehrenberg 2006; Li, Sloboda, and Vickers 2011). Epidemiological and animal studies have shown that pregnancies complicated by MS and obesity are at risk for premature cardiovascular disease, gestational diabetes, and preeclampsia and predispose the offspring to an increased risk of cardiovascular and metabolic disease later in life (Malek 2014; Chatzi, Plana, and Pappas 2009).

Maternal Interventions to Improve Offspring Outcomes in Rodent Models of Diet-Induced Obesity

Several interventions have been performed on animal models of metabolic diseases in pregnancy, in order to reduce maternal and fetal health issues.

A recent literature review looked at the studies testing those interventions administered either before pregnancy, throughout the entire gestation, or during gestation plus the lactation period (Menichini, Longo, and Facchinetti 2018).

Eight studies met the inclusion criteria. They have been performed in pregnancy after diet induced obesity (DIO) and have performed interventions in pregnancy with natural, synthetized compounds, and lifestyle modifications. Studies (Table 1) tested the efficacy of the following interventions:

- *Myo-inositol and D-chiro inositol*: the two main stereoisomers of the inositol family that play different roles as mediators of insulin. Their insulin-sensitizing activity by enhancing the glucose peripheral tissue uptake and glycogen synthesis has been demonstrated in rats, mouse, monkeys and humans (Croze and Soulage 2013).

- *Germinated brown rice (GBR) plus Gamma-Aminobutyric Acid (GABA) extract*: GBR is widely used in Asian countries (Imam and Ismail 2015), it possesses low glycemic load, therefore, promotes satiety and minimizes postprandial insulin secretion. In addition, the bioactive compounds present in GBR, named GABA, and oryzanol, mediate antiobesity effects through the regulation of peroxisome proliferator activated receptor-c (PPARc) gene. Other studies showed that prolonged consumption of GBR would result in a reduced weight gain during pregnancy (Imam MU 2014).
- *Resveratrol*: isolated from the oriental medicinal plant Polygonum capsidatum, it exerts a variety of anticancer and anti-inflammatory effects [19]. It also prevented adult hypertension, vascular dysfunction, and microvascular rarefaction in male offspring following in utero exposure to a low-protein diet (Bhat, Kosmeder, and Pezzuto 2001).
- *Exercise*: usually performed in mice/rats which are housed individually in cages equipped with running wheels or swimming activities. Maternal exercise has shown to have beneficial effects on offspring metabolic outcomes including improved glucose tolerance and increased glucose clearance in skeletal muscle and adipose tissue (Carter et al. 2012).
- *Adiponectin* (ADPN): an adipose tissue-derived hormone, involved in a wide variety of physiological processes, including energy metabolism, inflammation, and vascular physiology. It modulates the cross-talk between endothelial cells, smooth muscle cells, leukocytes, and platelets. ADPN exerts a vasoprotective action by enhancing the nitric oxide production and while decreasing ROS production in endothelial cells. In humans, plasma ADPN levels are positively associated with arterial vasodilation in response to nitroglycerine (a measure of endothelium-independent vasodilation) independent of insulin sensitivity (Vaiopoulos et al. 2012).

- *Taurine (2-aminoethanesulfonic acid):* a sulphonyl amino acid derived from methionine and cysteine metabolism and found ubiquitously in all mammalian tissues. Several studies have reported the effectiveness of taurine in treating insulin resistance (IR) (Anuradha and Balakrishnan 1999; Ito, Schaffer, and Azuma 2012). Taurine possesses a regulatory role on the glutamic acid decarboxylase (GAD), on neuronal calcium homeostasis and calcium-dependent processes, such as protein kinase C (PKC) activity (Nandhini, Thirunavukkarasu, and Anuradha 2005).

Among those interventions we will study in deep the effects of the combination of MI/DCI at the rate of 40:1, on pregnancy complicated by obesity and MS, analyzing also the subsequent effects of inositols supplementation on the offspring born to those dams.

Table 1. Pregnant Rodent Models (Menichini, Longo, and Facchinetti 2018)

Reference	Animal Model	Interventions
(Ferrari et al. 2016b) (Longo et al. 2017)	eNOS C57BL/6J on HFD (D12492, 60% of fat)	MI/DCI
(Vega et al. 2015) (Vega, Reyes-Castro, and Rodriguez-Gonzalez 2016)	Albino Wistar rats on HFD (23.5% protein, 20% animal lard, 5% fat, 21% polysaccharide, 21% simple sugars, 5% fiber, 3.5% mineral mix, 1% vitamin mix, energy 4.9 Kcal/g)	Resveratrol and Exercise
(Adamu et al. 2016)	Sprague Dawley rats on HFD (diet characteristics not specified)	Germinated Brown rice plus GABA extract
(Aye et al. 2015)	C57BL/6J mice on HFD (diet characteristics not specified)	Adiponectin
(Laker et al. 2014)	C57BL/6 mice on HFD (60% of fat)	Exercise
(Li et al. 2013)	Wistar rats on high fat and high fructose diet (20% protein, 45% fat, 35% carbohydrate, including 26% from fructose)	Taurine

MI and DCI play a key role in the insulin pathway, acting as insulin-sensitizing agents through the enhancement of glucose peripheral tissue uptake and glycogen synthesis (Larner 2002). *In vivo* animal (Croze and Soulage 2013; Croze, Géloën, and Soulage 2015) and human studies (Croze et al. 2013; Matarrelli, Vitacolonna, and D'Angelo 2013; Santamaria et al. 2015; D'Anna R, Scilipoti A, Giordano D 2013; D'Anna, Di Benedetto, and Scilipoti 2015) demonstrated that Inositols supplementation during pregnancy improve glucose profile and reduces the adverse effects of hyperglycemia.

METHODS

Mouse Models of Metabolic Syndrome and Obesity

Epidemiological studies have suggested that both the in utero environment and genetic factors play a fundamental role in the fetal origins of adult cardiovascular diseases (Huxley, Neil, and Collins 2002). To study these complex interactions, a transgenic mouse model lacking the endothelial nitric oxide synthase gene (NOS3), the rate-limiting enzyme responsible for nitric oxide (NO) production from L-arginine in endothelial cells, has been used (Furchgott 1984; Ignarro 1990). NO is a potent smooth muscle relaxant and an essential modulator of vascular tone (Rees et al. 1990); it also contributes to the maintenance of adequate uteroplacental perfusion through its vasodilatatory properties. Inhibition of NOS3 during pregnancy results in maternal hypertension and fetal growth restriction (Pallares and Gonzalez-Bulnes 2008; Tsukimori et al. 2008; Wagenseil et al. 2010). This animal model is well suited to study the contribution of each variable on fetal vascular programming and its long-term effects, as it combines an adverse uterine environment with a maternal genetic predisposition to abnormal vascular function (Chao-Yung and Liao 2012).

Metabolic-Like Syndrome Phenotype

Heterozygous mice lacking endothelial nitric oxide synthase (eNOS) gene and born to hypertensive mothers (Longo, Jain, and Vedernikov 2005), when fed high fat diet (HFD) develop metabolic like syndrome phenotype: obesity, glucose intolerance, elevated systolic blood pressure (SBP), low HDL, high insulin, and low adiponectin levels (Longo, Refuerzo, and Mann 2015).

Obesity Phenotype

Wild-type female mice when fed with an obesogenic diet (high fat diet, D12492, 60% of fat) for 4 consecutive weeks until 7-8 weeks of life, develop an obese phenotype (Chao-Yung and Liao 2012).

Inositols Administration during Pregnancy

The MI/DCI (40:1) mixture corresponds to the physiological plasma ratio of MI and DCI, which has been proven to be the most effective (Unfer and Porcaro 2014).

On gestational day 1, metabolic-like syndrome and obese mice were randomly allocated to receive either a mixture of MI/DCI dissolved in water, 7.2/0.18 mg/mL, respectively, based on animals (Croze and Soulage 2013; Croze, Géloën, and Soulage 2015) and human studies (Matarrelli et al. 2013; Santamaria et al. 2015; D'Anna, Di Benedetto, and Scilipoti 2015; Corrado, D'Anna, and Di Vieste 2011), or plain water as placebo. Considering that blood volume during pregnancy physiologically shows a 20% increase compared with the nonpregnant status, the MI/DCI doses have been adjusted by a 20% increase to the previously established doses used in a nonpregnant obese mouse model (MI: 6 mg/mL) (Croze, Géloën, and Soulage 2015).

The treatment was maintained until term gestation (gestational day 18 of pregnancy), when dams were sacrificed.

Pregnant mice were single housed to be able to carefully evaluate water intake and consequently the daily dose of MI/DCI. Daily water consumption was estimated by subtracting the total amount of water left in the bottle from the initial amount supplied. On average, pregnant mice drink 5 mL/day, so MI/DCI daily consumption was approximately 36/0.9 mg of, respectively, MI/DCI per day per mouse. At term gestation, the metabolic profile of the metabolic-like syndrome and obese pregnant dams were obtained including the following: SBP, a glucose tolerance test, maternal gestational weight gain, and serum levels of metabolic biomarkers relevant to diabetes and obesity. Dams were then killed, pups and placentas weights were collected (Ferrari et al. 2016b).

RESULTS

MI/DCI supplementation in pregnant mice with metabolic-like syndrome phenotype had improved blood pressure, glucose tolerance, and leptin levels. However, in obese pregnant mice, MI/DCI treatment prevented maternal increased weight gain associated with a high-fat diet but did not affect maternal glucose tolerance, blood pressure, and the metabolic markers related to diabetes.

These findings support the rationale for the use of combined MI/DCI supplementation in pregnancies complicated by MS but not by obesity alone in these animal models. Inositols are Food and Drug Administration approved supplements (Carlomagno and Unfer 2011) with a potential role in improving metabolic profile in MS. It is well established that MS, obesity and insulin resistance, during pregnancy have a negative impact on the pregnancy and on the metabolic and cardiovascular future health of the mother and the offspring (Catalano and Ehrenberg 2006; Li, Sloboda, and Vickers 2011; Malek 2014; Chatzi, Plana, and Pappas 2009; Kaul, Savu, and Nerenberg 2015).

Therefore, the potential of a new nonpharmacological approach as a preventive and therapeutic agent is clinically relevant because appropriate preventive strategies for MS in pregnancy have not yet been identified.

EFFECTS OF MATERNAL TREATMENT OF METABOLIC SYNDROME WITH INOSITOLS ON VASCULAR FUNCTION IN THE ADULT OFFSPRING

The effects of the combination of MI and DCI supplemented to pregnant dams affected by MS have been studied by Longo et al. in 2017.

As previously reported, the offspring exposed in utero to a perturbated environment develop cardiovascular and metabolic disease later in life (Malek 2014; Chatzi, Plana, and Pappas 2009). Thus, the offspring born to mothers who present a metabolic like syndrome phenotype, obtained using a transgenic mouse model lacking endothelial nitric oxide synthase (Longo, Jain, and Vedernikov 2005), present an altered vascular function and hypertension as adults, confirming that the abnormal uterine environment in which offspring develop, alters the fetal and postnatal growth, resulting in cardiovascular diseases later in life (Longo et al. 2016).

Longo et al. evaluated if inositol treatment in pregnancy complicated by MS improves vascular profile in offspring programmed in utero to develop hypertension.

They used a heterozygous eNOS-/+ mice fed a high fat diet which manifest a MS phenotype. Females eNOS-/+ with MS have been bred with wild type (WT), normotensive males to obtain a *pregnant mouse model of MS*. On gestational day 1 (GD1), dams were allocated to receive a mixture of inositols (MI/DCI: 7.2/0.18 mg/ml, at the rate of 40:1) or water as control until delivery.

The mothers with genotype eNOS-/+ (heterozygous) when cross-bred with a WT male, generate either genetically normal (WT) offspring, who didn't inherit the altered eNOS gene, and genetically modified offspring, heterozygous for eNOS gene (Figure 2).

Therefore, the offspring obtained were genotyped and categorized as: WT offspring (genetically normal, with eNOS +/+ gene) and eNOS-/+ (genetically modified, heterozygous for eNOS gene).

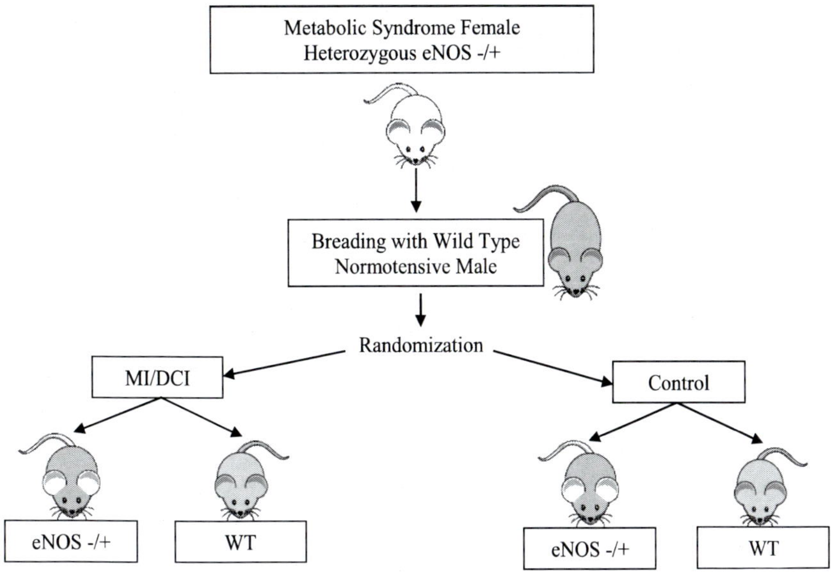

Figure 2. Scheme of the offspring born to Metabolic like syndrome mother and a normotensive mother, presenting either normal or altered genotype.

Both offspring developed in an abnormal uterine environment due to maternal MS. At 10 weeks of age, which correspond to adulthood, offspring SBP and vascular reactivity were evaluated.

Systolic Blood Pressure Measurement

SBP measurements were obtained using a calibrated, 8-chamber, tail-cuff system (CODA; Kent Scientific, Torrington, CT). Adult offspring were kept warm through a warming pad. Mice underwent an initial 10 cycles of acclimatization period; blood pressure was then monitored and recorded over 20 new cycles, which were averaged and used for the data analysis (Whitesall et al. 2004; Feng et al. 2008).

Vascular Reactivity Measurement

Carotid arteries were dissected from adult offspring for *in vitro*-vascular reactivity studies using a wire-myography system. The vessels were mounted in the chamber between two force transducers and bathed in Krebs solution at 37 degrees Celsius and pH of 7.4. The tension generated by the vascular tissue was recorded with a graduated micromanipulator and acquired by power lab computer software. Responses to the contractile agent, phenylephrine (PE), an α1 adrenergic agonist, in the presence and absence of a non-specific nitric oxide synthase inhibitor, NG-nitro-L-arginine methyl ester (L-NAME), were obtained. For the vasorelaxation responses, acetylcholine (ACh), an endothelium-dependent vasorelaxant agent, and sodium nitroprusside (SNP), an endothelium independent vasorelaxant agent, were evaluated.

SBP was significantly higher in eNOS-/+ offspring compared to the genetically normal WT, confirming that the genetic millieu plus an adverse uterine environment, result in hypertension development in adulthood.

Interestingly, the offspring who inherited the altered gene (eNOS-/+) born to MS mother treated with Inositols during pregnancy benefited more of maternal treatment than the genetically normal (WT) offspring, showing a significant decrease in SBP.

The altered uterine environment, resulted in an impaired vaso-relaxant response to Acetylcholine in both eNOS-/+ and WT offspring born to MS dams, showing that, vascular relaxation is affected by in utero perturbations, contrarily to what happened for the SBP. Surprisingly, maternal MI/DCI treatment improved the vascular relaxation in both the genetically normal and altered offspring. No differences were seen between the groups in the vasorelaxant responses to SNP.

Likewise, the contractile response to phenylephrine was higher in eNOS-/+ offspring compared to WT and was decreased by maternal Inositols treatment. No differences were seen in contractile response to L-NAME.

Inositol treatment improved SBP and vascular response in adult offspring born to dams with MS. Interestingly WT born to MS dams show an altered vascular profile similar to eNOS-/+ offspring and exhibit a higher response to Inositol treatment. These findings suggest that the benefits from MI and DCI treatment are limited to offspring exposed to environmental factors in-utero, and less likely in those due to genetic factors (Longo et al. 2017).

CONCLUSION

Cardiovascular and metabolic diseases are two of the main leading causes of death, worldwide. During the last century, an increase in the migration of rural populations to urban areas has led to significant dietary changes and an increased degree of obesity and metabolic disorders.

In evolutionary terms, fetal programming is not intended to help adults to survive longer but rather exists to provide a mechanism for the fetus to adapt to conditions in the intrauterine environment. Fetal programming predisposes people to certain adult diseases and is an important matter of concern in the current age of low fertility and an aging population because it suggests that the treatment of dysmetabolism (obesity and MS) during pregnancy can prevent many adult diseases.

According to the studies previously presented (Ferrari et al. 2016a; Longo et al. 2017), it seems that the supplementation with MI and DCI at the rate of 40:1 in pregnancy could ameliorate different components of metabolic and cardiovascular profile of both the mother and the offspring, in animal models of maternal obesity and MS.

Indeed, combined inositols treatment during pregnancy improved blood pressure, glucose levels at the glucose tolerance test and leptin levels in pregnant dams with a metabolic like syndrome phenotype and resulted to be associated with lower gestational weight gain in the obese pregnant dams.

Similar to what described in mice, inositol supplementation improved maternal glucose tolerance in many conditions of metabolic risk also in women, namely those with polycystic ovary syndrome (D'Anna R, Di Benedetto V, Rizzo P 2012). The early supplementation in pregnancy indeed provided efficacy in the prevention of gestational diabetes either in obese (D'Anna, Di Benedetto, and Scilipoti 2015) and in overweight women (Santamaria et al. 2015). Considering the beneficial effects showed by inositols supplementation during pregnancy in animals and humans, we are allowed to believe that they could prevent, as observed in animals, the intergenerational transmission of metabolic/vascular derangements, also in humans. It is, therefore, clear that a lot of different mechanisms participate in conditioning the metabolic fetal programing. Such mechanisms are likely due to the positive modulation of epigenetic changes associated with maternal obesity. Those processes could include the hypo-methylation of metabolic regulators, in the offspring, resulting in enhanced gene expression and preserved metabolic function later in life as well as, the amelioration and/or suppression of maternal dyslipidemia, glucose alteration, oxidative stress, and systemic inflammation, which results in a reconstitution of a favorable gestational environment (Nathanielsz et al. 2013; Menichini, Longo, and Facchinetti 2018).

MI/DCI treatment improved SBP and vascular response in adult offspring born to dams with MS. Interestingly, the genetically normal WT born to MS dams show an altered vascular profile similar to the genetically altered eNOS-/+ offspring and exhibit a higher response to inositols treatment. Thus, the findings presented suggest that the benefits from inositols treatment are limited to offspring exposed to environmental factors in-utero, and less likely in those due to genetic factors.

The epigenetic programming described occurs in response to an in-utero stress or "insults" such as maternal metabolic and cardiovascular disorders. Individuals with genetic susceptibilities may be the most vulnerable to the in-utero influences and the epigenetic programming can lead to altered gene expression and consequently abnormal in utero organ differentiation contributing to long-term metabolic and cardiovascular consequences. Additionally, as seen in the animal models above presented, the association of an abnormal in utero fetal metabolic programming with a genetically altered background can lead to an earlier and more severe manifestation of metabolic disease in adulthood (Longo et al. 2016) which results to be less likely to be reversible.

We are far from the translation of the above findings to guide clinical interventions. However, the experimental studies here reviewed indicate that clinical research could now start to explore the efficacy and safety of inositols supplementation during pregnancy, interrupting the vicious circle that a mother affected by obesity and MS generates a child prone to develop metabolic and cardiovascular disease in adult life.

Conflict of Interest

None.

References

Adamu, H. A., M. U. Imam, D. J. Ooi, N. M. Esa, R. Rosli, and M. Ismail. 2016. "Perinatal exposure to germinated brown rice and its gamma amino-butyric acid-rich extract prevents high fat dietinduced insulin resistance in first generation rat offspring." *Food Nutr Res*. 60(1):30209.

Anuradha, C., and S. Balakrishnan. 1999. "Taurine attenuates hypertension and improves insulin sensitivity in the fructose-fed rat, an animal model of insulin resistance." *Can J Physiol Pharmacol*. 77:749–754.

Aye, I., F. Rosario, T. L. Powell, and T. Jansson. 2015. "Adiponectin supplementation in pregnant mice prevents the adverse effects of maternal obesity on placental function and fetal growth." *Proc Natl Acad Sci USA*. 112(41):12858–12863.

Barker, D., C. Osmond, J. Golding, D. Kuh, and M. Wadsworth. 1989 "Growth in utero, blood pressure in childhood and adult life, and mortality from cardiovascular disease." *BMJ*. 298:564–567.

Barker, D. 1990. "The fetal and infant origins of adult disease." *BMJ*. 301(6761):1111.

Barker, D. 1995. "Fetal origins of coronary heart disease." *BMJ*. 311:171–4.

Barker, D. 1997. "Maternal nutrition, fetal nutrition, and disease in later life." *Nutrition*. 13:807–813.

Barker, D. 1998. "In utero programming of chronic disease." *Clin Sci*. 95:115–28.

Barker, D. Mothers, babies, and health in later life. In: *Edinburgh: Churchill Livingstone*. 1998.

Barker, D., A. Shiell, E. Barker, and M. Law. 2000. "Growth in utero and blood pressure levels in the next generation." *J Hypertens*. 18:843–846.

Benyshek, D. 2013. "The "early life" origins of obesity-related health disorders: new discoveries regarding the intergenerational transmission of developmentally programmed traits in the global cardiometabolic health crisis." *Am J Phys Anthr.* 152(57):79–93.

Bhat, K., J. Kosmeder, and J. Pezzuto. 2001. "Biological effects of resveratrol. Antioxid Redox Signal." *Antioxid Redox Signal.* 3(6):1041-64.

Carlomagno, G., and V. Unfer. 2011. "Inositol safety: clinical evidences." *Eur Rev Med Pharmacol Sci.* 15:931–6.

Carter, L., K. Lewis, D. Wilkerson, and E. Al. 2012. "Perinatal exercise improves glucose homeostasis in adult offspring." *Am J Physiol Endocrinol Metab.* 303:1061–1068.

Catalano, P. M., and H. M. Ehrenberg. 2006. "The short- and long-term implications of maternal obesity on the mother and her offspring." *BJOG.* 113(10):1126-33.

Chao-Yung, W. C., and J. Liao. 2012. "A mouse model of diet-induced obesity and insulin resistance." *Methods Mol Biol.* 821:421–33.

Chatzi, L., E. Plana, and A. Pappas. 2009. "The metabolic syndrome in early pregnancy and risk of gestational diabetes mellitus." *Diabetes Metab.* 35:490–4.

Chiossi, G., M. Costantine, E. Tamayo, G. Hankins, G. Saade, and M. Longo. 2016. "Fetal programming of blood pressure in a transgenic mouse model of altered intrauterine environment." *J Physiol.* 7015–7025.

Corrado, F., R. D'Anna, G. Di Vieste, D. Giordano, B. Pintaudi, A. Santamaria, and A. Di Benedetto. 2011. "The effect of myoinositol supplementation on insulin resistance in patients with gestational diabetes." *Diabet Med.* 28:972–5.

Croze, M. L., and C. O. Soulage. 2013. "Potential role and therapeutic interests of myo-inositol in metabolic diseases." *Biochimie.* 95(10):1811–27.

Croze, M. L., R. E. Vella, N. J. Pillon, H. A. Soula, L. Hadji, M. Guichardant, and C. O. Soulage. 2013. "Chronic treatment with myo-inositol reduces white adipose tissue accretion and improves insulin sensitivity in female mice." *J Nutr Biochem.* 24(2):457–66.

Croze, M. L., and A. S. C. Géloën. 2015. "Abnormalities in myo-inositol metabolism associated with type 2 diabetes in mice fed a high fat diet: benefits of a dietary myo-inositol supplementation." *Br J Nutr.* 113:1862-75.

Cunningham, S., and I. Cameron. 2003. "Consequences of fetal growth restriction during childhood and adult life." *Curr Obs Gynaecol.* 13:212–7.

D'Anna, R., V. Di Benedetto, P. Rizzo, E. Raffone, M. L. Interdonato, F. Corrado, and A. Di Benedetto. 2012. "Myo-inositol may prevent gestational diabetes in PCOS women." *Gynecol Endocrinol.* 28:440–2.

D'Anna, R., A. Scilipoti, D. Giordano, C. Caruso, M. L. Cannata, M. L. Interdonato, F. Corrado, and A. Di Benedetto. 2013. "Myo-Inositol supplementation and onset of gestational diabetes mellitus in pregnant women with a family history of type 2 diabetes: a prospective, randomized, placebo-controlled study." *Diabetes Care.* (36):854–7.

D'Anna, R., A. Di Benedetto, A. Scilipoti, A. Santamaria, M. L. Interdonato, E. Petrella, I. Neri, B. Pintaudi, F. Corrado, and F. Facchinetti. 2015. "Myo-inositol supplementation for prevention of gestational diabetes in obese pregnant women: a randomized controlled trial." *Obs Gynecol.* 126:310–5.

Feng, M., S. Whitesall, Y. Zhang, M. Beibel, L. D'Alecy, and K. Di Petrillo. 2008. "Validation of volumepressure recording tail-cuff blood pressure measurements." *Am J Hypertens.* 21:1288–91.

Ferrari, F., F. Facchinetti, A. E. Ontiveros, R. P. Roberts, M. M. Saade, S. C. Blackwell, B. M. Sibai, J. S. Refuerzo, and M. Longo. 2016. "The effect of combined inositol supplementation on maternal metabolic profile in pregnancies complicated by metabolic syndrome and obesity." *Am J Obstet Gynecol.* 215(4):503.e1-8.

Furchgott, R. 1984. "The role of endothelium in the responses of vascular smooth muscle to drugs." *Annu Rev Pharmacol Toxicol.* 24:175–197.

Godfrey, K. 2002. "The role of the placenta in fetal programming: a review." *Placenta.* 23(A):20–7.

Hutcheson, R., and P. Rocic. 2012. "The metabolic syndrome, oxidative stress, environment, and cardiovascular disease: the great exploration." *Exp Diabetes Res*. 271–8.

Huxley, R., A. Neil, and R. Collins. 2002. "Unravelling the fetal origins hypothesis: is there really an inverse association between birth weight and subsequent blood pressure?" *Lancet*. 360:659–665.

Ignarro, L. 1990. "Biosynthesis and metabolism of endothelium-derived nitric oxide." *Annu Rev Pharmacol Toxicol*. (30):535–560.

Imam, M. U., A. Ishaka, D. J. Ooi, N. D. Md Zamri, N. Sarega, M. Ismail, and N. M. Esa. 2014. "Germinated Brown Rice Regulates Hepatic Cholesterol Metabolism and Cardiovascular Disease Risk in Hypercholesterolaemic Rats." *J Funct Foods*. 8:193–203.

Imam, M., and M. Ismail. 2015. *An overview on germinated brown rice and its nutragenomic implications*. New York: Wiley. 504–17.

Ito, T., S. Schaffer, and J. Azuma. 2012. "The potential usefulness of taurine on diabetes mellitus and its complications." *Amino Acids*. 42(5):529–1539.

Kaul, P., A. Savu, K. A. Nerenberg, L. E. Donovan, C. L. Chik, E. A. Ryan, and J. A. Johnson. 2015. "Impact of gestational diabetesmellitus and high maternal weight on the development of diabetes, hypertension and cardiovascular disease: a population level analysis." *Diabet Med*. 32:164–73.

Laker, R. C., T. S. Lillard, M. Okutsu, M. Zhang, K. L. Hoehn, J. J. Connelly, and Z. Yan. 2014. "Exercise prevents maternal high-fat diet-induced hypermethylation of the Pgc-1a gene and age-dependent metabolic dysfunction in the offspring." *Diabetes*. 63(5):1605–1611.

Larner, J. 2002. "D-chiro-inositol: its functional role in insulin action and its deficit in insulin resistance." *Int J Exp Diabetes Res*. 3:47–60.

Li, M., D. Sloboda, and M. Vickers. 2011. "Maternal Obesity and Developmental Programming of Metabolic Disorders in Offspring : Evidence from Animal Models." *Exp Diabetes Res*. 2011:592408.

Li, M., Reynolds C., Sloboda D., C. Gray, and M. H. Vickers. 2013 "Effects of taurine supplementation on hepatic markers of inflammation and lipid metabolism in mothers and offspring in the setting of maternal obesity." *PLoS One*. 8(10):e76961.

Longo, M., V. Jain, Y. P. Vedernikov, R. Bukowski, R. E. Garfield, G. D. Hankins, G. D. Anderson, and G. R. Saade. 2005. "Fetal origins of adult vascular dysfunction in mice lacking endothelial nitric oxide synthase." *Am J Physiol Regul Integr Comp Physiol*. 288:1114–21.

Longo, M., J. Refuerzo, and L. Mann. 2015. "Effect of high fat diet on metabolic programming in offspring born to hypertensive mother." *Am J Obs Gynecol*. 212(S):32–3.

Longo, M., J. S. Refuerzo, L. Mann, M. Leon, H. N. Moussa, B. M. Sibai, and S. C. Blackwell. 2016. "Adverse Effect of High-Fat Diet on Metabolic Programming in Offspring Born to a Murine Model of Maternal Hypertension." *Am J Hypertens*. 29(12):1366–73.

Longo, M., M. Alrais, E. H. Tamayo, F. Ferrari, F. Facchinetti, J. R. Refuerzo, S. C. Blackwell, and B. M. Sibai. 2017. "Does maternal treatment of metabolic syndrome with Inositol improve vascular function in their adult offspring?" *Am J Obstet Gynecol*. 216(1):75–76.

Lucas, A. 1994. "Role of nutritional programming in determining adult morbidity." *Arch Dis Child*. 71:288–90.

Malek, A. 2014. "The impact of metabolic disease associated with metabolic syndrome on human pregnancy." *Curr Pharm Biotechnol*. 15:3–12.

Matarrelli, B., E. Vitacolonna, and M. D'Angelo. 2013. "Effect of dietary myo-inositol supplementation in pregnancy on the incidence of maternal gestational diabetes mellitus and fetal outcomes: a randomized controlled trial." *J Matern Fetal Neonatal Med*. 26:967–72.

Menichini, D., M. Longo, and F. Facchinetti. 2018. "Maternal interventions to improve offspring outcomes in rodent models of diet-induced obesity: a review." *J Matern Neonatal Med*. 1–10.

Nandhini, A., V. Thirunavukkarasu, and C. Anuradha. 2005. "Taurine modifies insulin signaling enzymes in the fructose-fed insulin resistant rats." *Diabetes Metab*. 31(4):337–344.

Nathanielsz, P. W., S. P. Ford, N. M. Long, C. C. Vega, L. A. Reyes-Castro, and E. Zambrano. 2013. "Interventions to prevent adverse fetal programming due to maternal obesity during pregnancy." *Nutr Rev.* 71:78–87.

Pallares, P., and A. Gonzalez-Bulnes. 2008 "Intrauterine growth retardation in endothelial nitric oxide synthase-deficient mice is established from early stages of pregnancy." *Biol Reprod.* 78:1002–1006.

Santamaria, A., A. Di Benedetto, E. Petrella, B. Pintaudi, F. Corrado, R. D'Anna, I. Neri, and F. Facchinetti. 2015. "Myo-inositol may prevent gestational diabetes onset in overweight women: a randomized, controlled trial." *J Matern Neonatal Med.* 1–4.

Tsukimori, K., H. Komatsu, K. Fukushima, T. Kaku, H. Nakano, and N. Wake. 2008. "Inhibition of nitric oxide synthetase at mid-gestation in rats is associated with increases in arterial pressure, serum tumor necrosis factor-alpha, and placental apoptosis." *Am J Hypertens.* 21:477–481.

Unfer, V., and G. Porcaro. 2014. "Updates on the myoinositol plus D-chiro-inositol combined therapy in polycystic ovary syndrome." *Expert Rev Clin Pharmacol.* 7:623–31.

Vaiopoulos, A., K. Marinou, C. Christodoulides, and M. Koutsilieris. 2012. "The role of adiponectin in human vascular physiology." *Int J Cardiol.* 155(2):188–93.

Vega, C. C., L. A. Reyes-Castro, C. J. Bautista, F. Larrea, P. W. Nathanielsz, and E. Zambrano. 2015. "Exercise in obese female rats has beneficial effects on maternal and male and female offspring metabolism." *Int J Obes.* 39(4):712–9.

Vega, C. C., L. A. Reyes-Castro, and G. Rodrıguez-Gonzalez. 2016. "Resveratrol partially prevents oxidative stress and metabolic dysfunction in pregnant rats fed a low protein diet and their offspring." *J Physiol.* 594(5):1483–1499.

Wagenseil, J., C. Ciliberto, R. Knutsen, M. Levy, A. Kovacs, and R. Mecham. 2010. "The importance of elastin to aortic development in mice." *Am J Physiol Hear Circ Physiol.* 299(H):257–264.

Whitesall, S., J. Hoff, A. Vollmer, and L. D'Alecy. 2004. "Comparison of simultaneous measurement of mouse systolic arterial blood pressure by radiotelemetry and tail-cuff methods." *Am J Physiol Hear Circ Physiol.* 286:2408–15.

Widdowson, E., and R. McCance. 1975. "A review: new thoughts on growth." *Pediatr Res*. 9:154–6.

In: Inositols
Editor: Vittorio Unfer
ISBN: 978-1-53614-912-8

Chapter 11

INOSITOLS IN GYNECOLOGIC ONCOLOGY

Simona Dinicola[1,*], PhD, Alessandra Cucina[2,3], PhD and Mariano Bizzarri[1], PhD

[1]Department of Experimental Medicine,
Sapienza University of Rome, Rome, Italy
[2]Department of Surgery "Pietro Valdoni,"
Sapienza University of Rome, Rome,Italy
[3]Azienda Policlinico Umberto I, Rome, Italy

ABSTRACT

Studies on myo-inositol (MI) are gaining momentum given the critical role they play in a number of diseases, including cancer. Namely, in different tumors, inositol content (including inositol hexakisphosphate, InsP6) and inositol-based pathways have been demonstrated to be significantly deregulated. On the other hand, inositols supplementation reduces cells growth by inhibiting pRB phosphorylation and consequently the pRB/E2F complexes formation, a key step during cell cycle progression. Inositol reduces PI3K levels, thus counteracting the activation of the PKC/RAS/ERK pathway downstream of PI3K activation. Upstream

* Corresponding Author's Email: simona.dinicola@uniroma1.it.

of that pathway, inositol disrupts the ligand interaction between FGF and its receptor as well as with the EGF-transduction processes involving IGF-II receptor and AP-1 complexes. Furthermore, inositol addition inhibits Akt activation, thus leading to NF-kB inhibition. Concomitantly, inositol downregulates inflammatory markers, like COX-2 and PGE2, as well as the expression of several genes, including presenilin-1(PS1) and Notch-1. These effects promote the reversion of the epithelial-mesenchymal transition (EMT), by reducing Wnt-activation, β-catenin translocation, Notch-1, N-cadherin and SNAI1 release. Inositols interfere also directly with cytoskeleton components, by up-regulating focal adhesion kinase and E-cadherin, and decreasing fascin and cofilin, leading hence to invasiveness inhibition. Ultimately, the inositol-induced impairment of metalloproteinases and ROCK1/2 further reinforces the negative modulation on cell motility. Overall, these effects enable inositols in remodeling cytoskeleton architecture and cell-microenvironment relationships.

Keywords: Myo-Inositol, Inositol hexakisphosphate, gynecological cancer, cytoskeleton, tumor microenvironment

ABBREVIATIONS

AP-1, activator protein 1; COX, cyclooxygenase; EGF, Epidermal growth factor; EGFR, epidermal growth factor receptor; ERK, extracellular signal-regulated protein kinase; FGF, fibroblast growth factors; IGF-I, Insulin-like growth factor 1; IGF-II, Insulin-like growth factor 2; ISYNA1, inositol-3-phosphate synthase 1; IPG, inositol-phosphoglycans; MAPK, mitogen-activated protein kinase; MMPs, metalloproteinases; mRNA, messenger ribonucleic acid; NF-κB, nuclear factor kappa-light-chain-enhancer of activated B cells; PGE2, prostaglandin E2; PGES, prostaglandin E synthase; PI3K, phosphatidylinositol-3-OH kinase; PS1, presenilin-1; PKC, Protein kinase C; Akt, Protein kinase B; ROCK, Rho-associated protein kinase; TGFβ, transforming growth factor-beta; p21, cyclin-dependent kinase inhibitor 1; p27, cyclin-dependent kinase inhibitor 1B p53, tumor protein p53; p57, cyclin-dependent kinase inhibitor 1C; VEGF, vascular endothelial growth factor

Introduction

MI is among the oldest component of living beings, undergoing complex evolutionary modifications ultimately leading to the current multiplicity of functions for inositol-containing molecules in eukaryotes (Bizzarri et al. 2016). Besides the biological role sustained in its free form, MI and its phosphate derivatives – chiefly represented by InsP6 - also serve as important components of structural lipids and secondary messengers.

Deregulation of inositol-based cellular pathways have been established in several pathological conditions (Bizzarri et al. 2016). Namely, both InsP6 and MI showed to play critical roles in both carcinogenesis and breast cancer development. Conversely, InsP6 and MI display significant chemopreventive effects *in vitro* and *in vivo*, as they modulate a number of processes, including mRNA transcription, chromatin remodeling, cytoskeleton configuration, p53 activity, just to mention a few. These new findings prompted reassessing under a new light the molecular mechanistic anticancer effect of inositols.

Molecular Mechanisms of Action

Cell Cycle Control and Apoptosis

Numerous studies have explored the inhibitory activity of inositols on cancer cells growth. Results show that InsP6 induces G1 phase arrest and shortens S phase of cancer cells, chiefly by modulation of cyclins. Moreover, inositols up-regulate p53, p57, p27 and p21, and down-regulate the phosphorylated form of pRB. InsP6, by increasing the hypophosphorylated form of pRB, increases pRB/E2F complexes formation, thus blocking further progression along the cell cycle (Vucenik et al. 2005). Furthermore, InsP6 reduces the expression of genes involved in cell cycle advancement, while increasing the activity of those involved in cell-cycle inhibition. Down-regulation of breast cancer proliferation has been shown to occur in both estrogen-positive and estrogen-negative cells (Shamsuddin, Yang, and Vucenik 1996). While early studies suggested that inositol effect is rather cytostatic than cytotoxic (Vucenik et al. 1998), it has been later showed that InsP6 actively induces apoptosis in several cancer cell lines (Ferry et al. 2002). Moreover, InsP6 synergizes with Doxorubicin and Tamoxifen in inducing apoptosis in drug-resistant cancer cell lines (Tantivejkul et al. 2003). However, MI has been shown having only a minimal pro-apoptotic activity, even if it significantly synergize with InsP6, both *in vitro* and *in vivo*, in inducing cancer inhibition (Vucenik and Shamsuddin 2003).

It is worth noting that cell culture conditions may alternatively trigger differentiating processes of cancer cells (Sakamoto, Venkatraman, and Shamsuddin 1993, Yang and Shamsuddin 1995). Why cancer cells respond so differently following Inositol administration is not yet clear. Probably, other factors (i.e., inositol phosphate derivatives) participate in such processes, so driving the final output into diverse fates (Pittet et al. 1989).

The p53 Network

Selective activation of p53 activity is a critical step in committing cells towards apoptosis or growth inhibition. It is noteworthy that InsP6 increases p53 levels several folds, at both mRNA and protein level (Węglarz et al. 2006), even if p53 is not mandatory for InsP6/MI pro-apoptotic activity, as both apoptosis and inhibition of cell growth have been both observed in cancer cells lacking p53 (Roy et al. 2009, Zhang et al. 2000). Activation of p53, in turn, increases the endogenous synthesis of MI through ISYNA1 gene modulation, thus reinforcing the apoptotic commitment through to a positive feedback loop (Koguchi et al. 2016). Furthermore, p53-dependent increase in intracellular MI synthesis is mandatorily required to sustain growth inhibition as well as for inhibiting chemotherapy-induced resistance in cancer cells (Koguchi et al. 2016). Downstream of p53, InsP6 reduces pro-survival factors and up-regulates caspases and other pro-apoptotic factors (Diallo et al. 2008), while in normal cells, addiction of either InsP6 or MI, did not induce any significant apoptotic effect. It is noteworthy that breast cancer cells show significantly reduced levels of MI, as documented by metabolomic studies (Beckonert et al. 2003).

Inhibition of the PI3K/Akt Pathway

The PI3K/Akt pathways is a pivotal hub, upstream the activation of many survival pathways. PI3K triggers the phosphorylation-dependent activation of Akt. In turn, activated Akt modulates the function of numerous substrates involved in the regulation of cell cycle progression, ultimately allowing cancer cells becoming more aggressive. Both InsP6 and MI significantly reduce PI3K expression (Liu et al. 2015) (at both mRNA and protein level) and Akt activation by inhibiting its phosphorylation (Dinicola et al. 2016, Huang et al. 1997). InsP6 impairs directly PI3K activity and the PI3K-dependent activation of the tumor promoter-induced AP-1, as well as the phosphorylation-dependent activation of ERK and other MAPK, both *in vitro* and *in vivo* (Gu et al. 2009, Han et al. 2009). Given that PI3K/Akt pathway activity is mandatory required for triggering EMT, blocking PI3K would hinder the transformation of cancer cells into a more aggressive phenotype. Indeed, breast cancer cells treated *in vitro* with MI showed increased E-cadherin, down-regulation of metalloproteinase-9, redistribution of β-catenin behind cell membrane, while motility and invading capacity were severely inhibited (Dinicola et al. 2016). Those changes were associated with the down-regulation of PI3K/Akt activity, leading to a decrease in downstream signaling effectors: NF-kB, COX-2, and SNAI1. Moreover, MI decreases PS1 levels and inhibits its activity, thus decreasing both Notch 1 and SNAI1 levels. Furthermore, InsP6 impairs NFkB in cancer cells, by inhibiting its activation or by preventing the nuclear translocation of NFkB and NFkB-luciferase transcription activity (Ferry et al. 2002). Those changes are associated with a dramatic cytoskeleton remodeling (Dinicola et al. 2016), thereby suggesting that MI inhibits the principal molecular pathway supporting EMT in breast cancer cells.

Inhibition of Invasiveness and Motility

MI significantly hampers both motility and invasiveness of breast cancer cells (Dinicola et al. 2016). This effect is due to cytoskeleton remodeling and the concomitant inhibition of MMPs release (Dinicola et al. 2016). Similarly, InsP6 significantly reduces the number of lung metastatic colonies in a mouse metastatic tumor model (Vucenik et al. 1992), while in MDA-MB-231 breast cancer cells, reduced MMPs release upon inositol addition, enhanced invasiveness inhibition (Tantivejkul, Vucenik, and Shamsuddin 2003).

Wnt Signaling and Anti-Inflammatory Effects

Overexpression of the Wnt ligand – usually in association with deregulated γ-secretase activity - may lead to altered expression and redistribution of β-catenin and of several molecular factors belonging to the so-called inflammatory pathway, like COX-2 and PGE2. Increased expression of the aforementioned molecules has been associated with carcinogenesis in numerous tissues, chiefly in colon cancer (Luu et al. 2004). InsP6 down-regulates both *in vitro* and *in vivo* the Wnt pathway via β-catenin inhibition, hence significantly reducing COX-2 at the mRNA and protein level (Shafie et al. 2013). Similarly, in breast cancer cells MI has proven to down-regulate both NF-kB and COX-2, while relocating β-catenin behind cell membrane and inhibiting its nuclear translocation (Dinicola et al. 2016). Inhibition on inflammatory markers is not limited to epithelial cells, as inositol activity also interferes with the pro-inflammatory activity of stroma cells. Indeed, both InsP6 and MI has demonstrated to prevent pulmonary fibrosis, breast density and chronic inflammatory damage, likely by influencing the cross talk among cells and their milieu (Kamp et al. 1995, Liao et al. 2007). Additionally, MI modulates the expression of both TGFβ and its receptors, thus mitigating its pro-inflammatory effects (Węglarz et al. 2006). Furthermore, InsP6 has been show to exert valuable effects on fibroblasts by blocking the syndecan-4 dependent focal adhesion and microfilament bound (Couchman et al. 2002). Syndecan-4, a heparan sulphate proteoglycan embedded into cellular membranes where it regulates cell-matrix interactions, binds to the FGF, fostering its coupling with the FGF receptor. InsP6 disrupts such interaction, thus preventing the FGF-based signaling (Morrison et al. 1994). Additionally, inositol-related effects on the cell microenvironment involve modulation of angiogenesis. Formation of new blood vessels is required for sustaining cancer growth and invasiveness. Disruption of the structural relationships among cancer cells and their microenvironment promotes neo-angiogenesis, mainly through the release of VEGF and basic FGF. InsP6 negatively modulates both VEGF and bFGF release from tumor cells and impairs endothelial cells growth (Vucenik et al. 2004). Reduced synthesis of VEGF may be likely due to InsP6-mediated inhibition on PI3K/Akt and MAPK/ERK pathways, given that both of them modulate VEGF up-regulation (Vucenik et al. 1992). Furthermore, the synergistic activity of hypoxia and IGF-II increases VEGF mRNA expression and up-regulates IGF-1 protein that, in turn, reinforces VEGF release. Given that InsP6 has been shown to antagonize IGF-II activity by inhibiting the IGF-II receptor binding (Kar, Quirion, and Parent 1994), it is probable that some InsP6 anti-angiogenic effects can be ascribed to this mechanism.

Overall, these data suggest that inositol and its phosphate derivatives exert several anti-cancer effects by interfering with numerous key biochemical pathways.

Anticancer Activity through Insulin Modulation

MI, as well as its isomer D-chiro-inositol (DCI), participate in both insulin and glucose metabolism, and deregulated MI metabolism has been documented in several conditions associated with diabetes or insulin resistance (Bizzarri et al. 2016). When insulin binds to its receptor, two distinct IPGs, incorporating either MI or DCI, are released by insulin-stimulated hydrolysis of glycosyl-phosphatidylinositol lipids located on the outer leaflet of the cell membrane. IPGs affect intracellular metabolic processes, namely by activating key enzymes controlling the oxidative and non-oxidative metabolism of glucose. Given that MI may efficiently counteract insulin resistance and its metabolic complications (D'Anna et al. 2015), it is tempting to speculate that it may also prevent IGF-I increase associated to those conditions. In turn, insulin resistance and increased levels of IGF-I are frequently associated with cancer and it is therefore conceivable that MI modulation of insulin activity may efficiently contribute in reducing tumor risk. Indeed, InsP6 has been already shown to inhibit the IGF-I/IGF-II receptor pathway-mediated sustained growth in cancer cells (Kar, Quirion, and Parent 1994, Tantivejkul, Vucenik, and Shamsuddin 2003).

Antioxidant and Other Effects

MI displays an appreciable anti-oxidant activity, while InsP6 is among the strongest anti-oxidants present in nature. By chelating polyvalent cations, InsP6 and MI suppress the Fenton reaction and the consequent release of hydroxyl radicals (Graf and Eaton 1990). In biological tissues, InsP6 inhibits Xanthine oxidase and reactive oxygen species production, thus dramatically inhibiting the free radical-based damage occurring in cells and tissues following inflammation, hypoxia or exposition to radiation injury (Rao et al. 1991). MI counteracts oxidative damage in fish exposed to environmental stresses and significantly inhibits systemic markers of oxidative stress in gynecological patients (Bizzarri et al. 2016). InsP6 scavenges superoxide radicals *in vitro* and *in vivo*, thus preventing formation of ADP-iron-oxygen complexes that trigger lipid peroxidation. Indeed, after InsP6 administration lipid peroxidation is significantly inhibited (Porres et al. 1999). As an increase in both reactive oxygen species and lipid peroxidation have been associated with cancer development, the anti-oxidant capabilities of InsP6 and MI could account for their anticancer chemopreventive effects.

Chemopreventive and Therapeutic Efficacy in Human Clinical Trials

Only a few pilot studies have been performed in order to ascertain the usefulness of inositols in clinical setting. InsP6 plus MI treatment of colon cancer patients is associated with appreciable reduction in tumor burden and improved quality of life (Druzijanic et al. 2002). Furthermore, significant longer survival and better quality of life have been obtained in breast and lung cancer patients treated with InsP6 and MI (Bačić et al. 2010). Moreover, Inositol ameliorates the responsiveness to antitumor drugs in breast cancer patients and markedly reduces incidence and severity of side effects (Bačić et al. 2010). As previously noticed in animal studies, MI exerts a significant chemopreventive activity also in humans. A study enrolling 26 smokers showed that MI in a daily dose up to 18 g/p.o. is safe and well tolerated, while inducing a significant regression of individual pulmonary dysplastic lesions (91% in the inositol-treated group versus 48% in control group) in a sample of heavy smoker individuals (Lam et al. 2006). This effect is probably linked to the observed inhibition of PI3K activity in dysplastic lesions.

Conclusion

MI and InsP6 play major biological functions, including modulation of cell cycle progression, apoptosis and differentiation. Evidence is mounting that inositol acts on both cytosolic and nuclear targets in enabling cells to successfully copy with many different stressor, namely during developmental processes and cellular differentiation (Bizzarri et al. 2016). Cancer is a kind of 'development gone awry,' in which the deregulation in the cross talk among cells and their microenvironment plays a relevant role. Given that inositol participates in the cell-stroma interplay, by modulating MMPs, E-cadherin, focal kinase complexes, and many other cytoskeletal components, it can be hypothesized that inositol and its derivatives may counteract cancer-related processes by specifically acting at this level, i.e., by restoring a 'normal' cell-stroma relationship. A recent paper, indeed, strongly support this hypothesis. In fact, InsP6 and MI prevent the development and metastatic progression of colon cancer in mice by modifying extracellular matrix proteins (collagen IV, fibronectin and laminin), integrin-1, matrix metalloproteinase 9, as well as several growth factors (VEGF, bFGF, TgFβ) (Fu et al. 2016).

Studies in this field are warranted in order to deepen our understanding of inositol mechanisms in both cancer and diseases of the development.

Conflict of Interest

None.

References

Bačić, Ivan, Nikica Družijanić, Robert Karlo, Ivan Škifić, and Stjepan Jagić. 2010. "Efficacy of IP 6+ inositol in the treatment of breast cancer patients receiving chemotherapy: prospective, randomized, pilot clinical study." *Journal of Experimental & Clinical Cancer Research* 29 (1):12.

Beckonert, Olaf, Jürgen Monnerjahn, Ulrich Bonk, and Dieter Leibfritz. 2003. "Visualizing metabolic changes in breast- cancer tissue using 1H- NMR spectroscopy and self- organizing maps." *NMR in Biomedicine: An International Journal Devoted to the Development and Application of Magnetic Resonance in vivo* 16 (1):1-11.

Bizzarri, M., A. Fuso, S. Dinicola, A. Cucina, and A. Bevilacqua. 2016. "Pharmacodynamics and pharmacokinetics of inositol(s) in health and disease." *Expert Opin Drug Metab Toxicol* 12 (10):1181-96. doi: 10.1080/17425255.2016.1206887.

Couchman, John R., Susan Vogt, Ssang-Taek Lim, Yangmi Lim, Eok-Soo Oh, Glenn D. Prestwich, Anne Theibert, Weontae Lee, and Anne

Woods. 2002. "Regulation of inositol phospholipid binding and signaling through syndecan-4." *Journal of Biological Chemistry* 277 (51):49296-303.

D'Anna, Rosario, Antonino Di Benedetto, Angela Scilipoti, Angelo Santamaria, Maria Lieta Interdonato, Elisabetta Petrella, Isabella Neri, Basilio Pintaudi, Francesco Corrado, and Fabio Facchinetti. 2015. "Myo-inositol supplementation for prevention of gestational diabetes in obese pregnant women: a randomized controlled trial." *Obstetrics & Gynecology* 126 (2):310-315.

Diallo, J. S., B. Betton, N. Parent, B. Peant, L. Lessard, C. Le Page, R. Bertrand, A. M. Mes-Masson, and F. Saad. 2008. "Enhanced killing of androgen-independent prostate cancer cells using inositol hexakisphosphate in combination with proteasome inhibitors." *British Journal of Cancer* 99 (10):1613.

Dinicola, Simona, Gianmarco Fabrizi, Maria Grazia Masiello, Sara Proietti, Alessandro Palombo, Mirko Minini, Abdel Halim Harrath, Saleh H. Alwasel, Giulia Ricci, and Angela Catizone. 2016. "Inositol induces mesenchymal-epithelial reversion in breast cancer cells through cytoskeleton rearrangement." *Experimental Cell Research* 345 (1):37-50.

Druzijanic, N., J. Juricic, Z. Perko, and D. Kraljevic. 2002. "IP-6 and Inositol: adjuvant to chemotherapy of colon cancer. A pilot clinical trial." *Rev Oncol* 4:171.

Ferry, Sandra, Miho Matsuda, Hiroki Yoshida, and Masato Hirata. 2002. "Inositol hexakisphosphate blocks tumor cell growth by activating apoptotic machinery as well as by inhibiting the Akt/NFκB-mediated cell survival pathway." *Carcinogenesis* 23 (12):2031-2041.

Fu, Min, Yang Song, Zhaoxia Wen, Xingyi Lu, and Lianhua Cui. 2016. "Inositol hexaphosphate and inositol inhibit colorectal cancer metastasis to the liver in BALB/c mice." *Nutrients* 8 (5):286.

Graf, Ernst, and John W. Eaton. 1990. "Antioxidant functions of phytic acid." *Free Radical Biology and Medicine* 8 (1):61-69.

Gu, Mallikarjuna, Srirupa Roy, Komal Raina, Chapla Agarwal, and Rajesh Agarwal. 2009. "Inositol hexaphosphate suppresses growth and induces apoptosis in prostate carcinoma cells in culture and nude mouse xenograft: PI3K-Akt pathway as potential target." *Cancer Research* 69 (24):9465-72.

Han, Wei, Joell J. Gills, Regan M. Memmott, Stephen Lam, and Phillip A. Dennis. 2009. "The chemopreventive agent myoinositol inhibits Akt and extracellular signal-regulated kinase in bronchial lesions from heavy smokers." *Cancer Prevention Research* 2 (4):370-6.

Huang, Chuanshu, Wei-Ya Ma, Stephen S. Hecht, and Zigang Dong. 1997. "Inositol hexaphosphate inhibits cell transformation and activator protein 1 activation by targeting phosphatidylinositol-3′ kinase." *Cancer Research* 57 (14):2873-2878.

Kamp, David W., Vatche A. Israbian, Anjana V. Yeldandi, Ralph J. Panos, Philip Graceffa, and Sigmund A. Weitzman. 1995. "Phytic acid, an iron chelator, attenuates pulmonary inflammation and fibrosis in rats after intratracheal instillation of asbestos." *Toxicologic Pathology* 23 (6):689-695.

Kar, S., R. Quirion, and A. Parent. 1994. "An interaction between inositol hexakisphosphate (IP6) and insulin-like growth factor II receptor binding sites in the rat brain." *Neuroreport* 5 (5):625-628.

Koguchi, Tomoyuki, Chizu Tanikawa, Jinichi Mori, Yoshiyuki Kojima, and Koichi Matsuda. 2016. "Regulation of myo-inositol biosynthesis by p53-ISYNA1 pathway." *International Journal of Oncology* 48 (6):2415-2424.

Lam, Stephen, Annette McWilliams, Calum MacAulay, Lee Wattenberg, and Eva Szabo. 2006. "A phase I study of myo-inositol for lung cancer chemoprevention." *Cancer Epidemiology and Prevention Biomarkers* 15 (8):1526-1531.

Liao, Jie, Darren N. Seril, Allison L. Yang, Gary G. Lu, and Guang-Yu Yang. 2007. "Inhibition of chronic ulcerative colitis associated adenocarcinoma development in mice by inositol compounds." *Carcinogenesis* 28 (2):446-454.

Liu, Guiyuan, Yang Song, Lianhua Cui, Zhaoxia Wen, and Xiaoqing Lu. 2015. "Inositol hexaphosphate suppresses growth and induces apoptosis in HT-29 colorectal cancer cells in culture: PI3K/Akt pathway as a potential target." *International Journal of Clinical and Experimental Pathology* 8 (2):1402.

Luu, Hue H., Ruiwen Zhang, Rex C. Haydon, Elizabeth Rayburn, Quan Kang, Weike Si, Jong K. Park, Hui Wang, Ying Peng, and Wei Jiang. 2004. "Wnt/β-catenin signaling pathway as novel cancer drug targets." *Current Cancer Drug Targets* 4 (8):653-671.

Morrison, Richard S., Ergang Shi, Mikio Kan, Fumio Yamaguchi, Wallace McKeehan, Maria Rudnicka-Nawrot, and Krzysztof Palczewski. 1994. "Inositolhexakisphosphate (Ins P 6): An antagonist of fibroblast growth factor receptor binding and activity." *In Vitro Cellular & Developmental Biology-Animal* 30 (11):783-789.

Pittet, Didier, Werner Schlegel, Daniel P. Lew, Antoinette Monod, and G. W. Mayr. 1989. "Mass changes in inositol tetrakis-and pentakisphosphate isomers induced by chemotactic peptide stimulation in HL-60 cells." *Journal of Biological Chemistry* 264 (31):18489-18493.

Porres, Jesús M., Chad H. Stahl, Wen-Hsing Cheng, Yangxin Fu, Karl R. Roneker, Wilson G. Pond, and Xin Gen Lei. 1999. "Dietary intrinsic phytate protects colon from lipid peroxidation in pigs with a moderately high dietary iron intake." *Proceedings of the Society for Experimental Biology and Medicine* 221 (1):80-86.

Rao, Parinam S., Xuekun Liu, Dipak K. Das, Gerald S. Weinstein, and Denis H. Tyras. 1991. "Protection of ischemic heart from reperfusion injury by myo-inositol hexaphosphate, a natural antioxidant." *The Annals of Thoracic Surgery* 52 (4):908-912.

Roy, Srirupa, Mallikarjuna Gu, Kumaraguruparan Ramasamy, Rana P. Singh, Chapla Agarwal, Sunitha Siriwardana, Robert A. Sclafani, and Rajesh Agarwal. 2009. "p21/Cip1 and p27/Kip1 are essential molecular targets of inositol hexaphosphate for its antitumor efficacy against prostate cancer." *Cancer Research* 69 (3):1166-1173.

Sakamoto, Kosaku, Giridhar Venkatraman, and Abulkalam M. Shamsuddin. 1993. "Growth inhibition and differentiation of HT-29 cells *in vitro* by inositol hexaphosphate (phytic acid)." *Carcinogenesis* 14 (9):1815-1819.

Shafie, Nurul Husna, Norhaizan Mohd Esa, Hairuszah Ithnin, Abdah Md Akim, Norazalina Saad, and Ashok Kumar Pandurangan. 2013. "Preventive inositol hexaphosphate extracted from rice bran inhibits colorectal cancer through involvement of Wnt/β-catenin and COX-2 pathways." *BioMed Research International* 2013.

Shamsuddin, Abulkalam M., Guang Yu Yang, and Ivana Vucenik. 1996. "Novel anti-cancer functions of IP6: growth inhibition and differentiation of human mammary cancer cell lines *in vitro*." *Anticancer Research* 16 (6A):3287-3292.

Tantivejkul, Kwanchanit, Ivana Vucenik, Julie Eiseman, and AbulKalam M. Shamsuddin. 2003. "Inositol hexaphosphate (IP 6) enhances the anti-proliferative effects of adriamycin and tamoxifen in breast cancer." *Breast Cancer Research and Treatment* 79 (3):301-312.

Tantivejkul, Kwanchanit, Ivana Vucenik, and Abulkalam M. Shamsuddin. 2003. "Inositol Hexaphosphate (IP 6) Inhibits Key Events of Cancer Metastasis: I. *In Vitro* Studies of Adhesion, Migration and Invasion of MDA-MB 231 Human Breast Cancer Cells." *In vivo* 23 (5A):3671-9.

Vucenik, I., T. Kalebic, K. Tantivejkul, and A. M. Shamsuddin. 1998. "Novel anticancer function of inositol hexaphosphate: inhibition of human rhabdomyosarcoma *in vitro* and *in vivo*." *Anticancer Research* 18 (3A):1377-1384.

Vucenik, I., A. Passaniti, M. I. Vitolo, K. Tantivejkul, P. Eggleton, and A. M. Shamsuddin. 2004. "Anti-angiogenic activity of inositol hexaphosphate (IP6)." *Carcinogenesis* 25 (11):2115-23. doi: 10.1093/carcin/bgh232.

Vucenik, Ivana, Gayatri Ramakrishna, Kwanchanit Tantivejkul, Lucy M. Anderson, and Danica Ramljak. 2005. "Inositol hexaphosphate (IP6) blocks proliferation of human breast cancer cells through a PKCδ-dependent increase in p27Kip1 and decrease in retinoblastoma protein (pRb) phosphorylation." *Breast Cancer Research and Treatment* 91 (1):35-45. doi: 10.1007/s10549-004-6456-5.

Vucenik, Ivana, and AbulKalam M. Shamsuddin. 2003. "Cancer inhibition by inositol hexaphosphate (IP6) and inositol: from laboratory to clinic." *The Journal of Nutrition* 133 (11):3778S-3784S.

Vucenik, Ivana, Vesna J. Tomazic, Dagmar Fabian, and Abulkalam M. Shamsuddin. 1992. "Antitumor activity of phytic acid (inositol hexaphosphate) in murine transplanted and metastatic fibrosarcoma, a pilot study." *Cancer Letters* 65 (1):9-13.

Węglarz, Ludmiła, Izabela Molin, Arkadiusz Orchel, Beata Parfiniewicz, and Zofia Dzierżewicz. 2006. "Quantitative analysis of the level of p53 and p21WAF1 mRNA in human colon cancer HT-29 cells treated with inositol hexaphosphate." *Acta Biochimica Polonica* 53 (2):349-56.

Yang, G. Y., and A. M. Shamsuddin. 1995. "IP6-induced growth inhibition and differentiation of HT-29 human colon cancer cells: involvement of intracellular inositol phosphates." *Anticancer Research* 15 (6B):2479-2487.

Zhang, Zhongqiu, Qing Liu, Laura E. Lantry, Yian Wang, Gary J. Kelloff, Marshall W. Anderson, Roger W. Wiseman, Ronald A. Lubet, and Ming You. 2000. "A germ-line p53 mutation accelerates pulmonary tumorigenesis: p53-independent efficacy of chemopreventive agents green tea or dexamethasone/myo-inositol and chemotherapeutic agents taxol or adriamycin." *Cancer Research* 60 (4):901-907.

In: Inositols
Editor: Vittorio Unfer

ISBN: 978-1-53614-912-8

Chapter 12

Associations of Inositol with Other Substances: Opportunity or Risks?

Fedele Manna*

Pharmaceutical and Toxicological Chemistry,
University of Rome LA SAPIENZA, Rome, Italy

Abstract

Inositol, and in particular myo-inositol (MI), is considered an essential dietary factor and its deficiency has been linked to several syndromes. After oral intake of inositol (by means of food or dietary supplements), its absorption takes place at intestinal level: notably, inositol transport occurs through the apical membranes of intestinal epithelia and it is then reabsorbed from the renal tubule lumen. Inositols' transport occurs through two main families of transport proteins: sodium ion coupled and proton coupled inositol. The sodium-dependent transporter SMIT2, responsible for intestinal inositol absorption, transports MI with an affinity constant (Km) of 120 μM as well as D-chiro-inositol (DCI) (Km = 130μM). Based on this evidence, it is possible to speculate that the intake of high doses of DCI may impair MI absorption.

* Associate Professor; Email: fedelemanna42@gmail.com.

Inositol intake during meals may result in the intestinal copresence of substances that may cause a marked decrease in inositol absorption. A similar limitation can occurr in inositol-based food supplements, in which the copresence of specific excipients may cause a reduction of inositol absorption due to interactions and/or competition for the same transporters. On the contrary, recent evidences suggest that the combined intake of MI and alpha-lactalbumin provides an enhanced MI bioavailability: further experiments should be performed in order to prove the mechanism of action and eventually identify further substances able to positively affect intestinal inositol absorption or give rise to additive/synergic pharmacological effects.

Keywords: inositol, transporter, pharmacokinetic, absorption

INTRODUCTION

Inositol (Ins) is among the oldest component of living beings, undergoing complex evolutionary modifications ultimately leading to the current multiplicity of functions for inositol-containing molecules in eukaryotes. Besides the biological role sustained in its free form, Ins also serves as an important component of structural lipids and of secondary messengers. Ins has structural resemblance to glucose and plays a pivotal role in many cellular and tissue processes, including development, metabolism regulation and regenerative medicine. It has been widely studied in the last decades when the interest of Ins is largely increased in several fields. Although being the most abundant form in nature, myo-inositol (MI) is only one of nine possible structural isomers of inositol, as other naturally occurring stereoisomers have been found: scyllo-, muco-, epi, neo-, allo-, cis-, D-chiro-and L-chiro-inositol. Among the nine isomers, only a few of those display significant physiological functions. Indeed, the MI moiety is widely utilized by nature to biosynthesize several intermediate molecular components of the biochemical machinery, including inositol phosphates (IPs or InPs), phosphatidylinositol (PI), phosphatidylinositides (phosphatidylinositol-phosphates PIPs or PtdIns), glycosylphosphatidylinositols (GPI), and many other derivatives as inositolphosphoglycans (IPG) and inositol ethers and esters. Beside MI, also D-chiro-inositol (DCI) has been reported as another important stereoisomer of MI particularly present in fat, muscle and liver tissues. In tissues, the physiological distribution of MI and DCI, which also influences their distinct physiological functions, is dependent by the enzymatic action of an epimerase which convert MI in DCI (Bizzarri et al. 2016).

MI occupies a central position in cellular metabolism and it is present in a wide variety of foods and food products at low concentrations. MI is associated with glucose transporters activation and glucose utilization, while DCI is mainly involved in the synthesis of glycogen in the liver, fat and muscle tissues. So far, several experimental and clinical studies have reported MI and DCI as second messengers of insulin in many insulin dependent processes that are involved in pathological conditions such as PCOS, diabetes mellitus type 2 and metabolic syndrome. MI and DCI consistently improve glucose metabolic markers, insulin resistance and dyslipidaemia (Chukwuma, Ibrahim, and Islam 2016).

MI also acts as a compatible osmolyte when cells are challenged by variation in extracellular tonicity. MI homeostasis in cells and tissue is maintained at three different levels: 1) intestinal absorption and renal excretion; 2) carrier-mediated transport across the plasma membrane; 3) endogenous synthesis and catabolism (Bizzarri et al. 2016).

It is well known that oral absorption of Ins, in particular MI, can be influenced by a variety of factors such as the physiochemical properties, formulation and dose of the compound, as well as the physiology and pathology of the gastrointestinal tract (GIT). In general terms, common approaches used to enhance drug and/or nutrients oral absorption are based on the chemical modification of the molecule in form of salt or prodrug and/or on the use of specifically designed pharmaceutical forms (gastro-resistent tablets, softgels, etc.) (Carlomagno et al. 2012).

Independently from the pharmaceutical form, after oral intake, Ins' absorption occurs at intestinal level and selective proteins are involved in its uptake. Notably, Ins transport occurs through the apical membranes of intestinal epithelia and renal proxila tube since it is both absorbed from dietary sources and reabsorbed from the renal tubule lumen (Bissonnette, Coady, and Lapointe 2004).

Ins intake during meals may result in the intestinal compresence of different sugars that may compete for or interfere with the same transporters, causing a marked decrease in inositol absorption. Similarly, in inositol-based drugs or food supplements, the combined presence of sugary excipients such as maltodextrin, sucrose, galactose, etc. may be responsible of a reduction of inositol absorption due to interactions and/or competition for the same transporters (Unfer 2018).

INOSITOL TRANSPORT PROTEINS

Ins transporters are responsible for uptake and intracellular distribution of Ins: they have been identified and studied in protozoa, bacteria, plants and animal. With specific reference to MI, clinical pharmacokinetic studies reported that its plasma concentration is about 20-30 μmol/l and originates from both dietary intake and synthesis from glucose (Carlomagno et al. 2012, De Grazia et al. 2012, Monastra et al. 2018). Compared to plasma concentration, intracellular content of MI is quite high (up to 30 mM): to achieve such high concentration of this polyol cells rely on cotransporters. Accumulation of MI within cells against its concentration gradient is accomplished by cotrasport, using the electrochemical gradient of the coupled ion.

Alteration in the transport and metabolism of MI are associated with several pathological conditions such as Down's syndrome, psychiatric disorders (i.e., depression, panic disorders, obsessive compulsive disorder), Alzheimer's disease, respiratory distress syndrome, cancer, metabolic syndrome and polycystic ovary syndrome for which clinical trials and, in some cases, metanalysis based on MI treatments were carried out and published (Baillargeon et al. 2008, Bizzarri et al. 2016). Several transport mechanisms are involved in the active uptake of MI into various types of cells.

In general terms, Ins transporters can be divided in two main families according to their transport mechanisms: sodium ion coupled and proton coupled inositol. Currently, three MI cotransporters have been identified: two are Na+-dependent (SMIT1 and SMIT2) and one is H+-dependent (HMIT) and predominantly expressed in the brain (Lahjouji et al. 2007).

SMIT1: Expression and Activities

The so-called SMIT1, namely sodium/MI transporter 1, was first identified in 1992 by Kwon et al. from Madin–Darby canine kidney (MDCK) cells, as the transporter responsible for accumulation of MI in kidney cells exposed to hypertonic medium (Kwon et al. 1992) and soon found also in rat, mouse and human. The protein was characterized in *Xenopus* oocytes and showed strong similarity with the Na-glucose cotransporter (SGLT) family.

At this regard, seven SGLT isoforms have been described so far (table 1) and SMIT1 is considered as isoform of this family (Van Steenbergen et al. 2017). The respective gene for SMIT1, *SLC5A3,* belongs to the Solute Carrier Family 5 (SLC5) which consists of eleven members in humans. Preferred substrate of SMIT1 is MI ($K_m = 55\ \mu M$) and *scillo*-inositol showed a similar affinity while only a very low affinity for glucose has been demonstrated ($K_m \sim 50$ mM). In competitive experiments, L-fucose was shown to inhibit in high concentration MI transport. SMIT1 is distributed in brain, heart, kidney and lung at plasma membranes level. It is the main actor in mammalian osmoregulation by accumulating MI in kidney and brain. The expression of the SLC5A3 is upregulated under hypertonic stress and high osmolality. Hypertonicity-induced expression of SLC5A3 is regulated by the transcription factor TonEBP (Tonicity-responsive Enhancer Binding Protein). TonEBP expression itself is upregulated under hypertonic conditions, resulting in an increased amount of TonEBP protein and its translocation to the nucleus.

The potential role of SMIT1 in Down syndrome, Alzheimer's disease and bipolar disorders has been investigated. The gene SLC5A3 is located on band q22 on chromosome 21 and Down syndrome is a genetic disorder caused by an extra chromosome 21. Subjects affected by this syndrome have shown elevated concentrations of MI in brain and cerebrospinal fluid that can already be detected in foeti during pregnancy. Down syndrome individuals affected by Alzheimer's disease (AD) are characterized by even higher levels of MI: this evidence implicates a possible role for SMIT1 also in AD. On the other hand, MI may also be helpful against AD: on this regard, more specific evidences have been reported on *scillo*-inositol which is imported in brain cells by SMIT1 and showed to inhibit the formation of amyloid β in mouse models.

Mice in which SMIT1 was genetically removed demonstrated the critical importance of MI transporter during development as the mice died soon after birth due to respiratory failure, although neonatal lethality could be prevented by prenatal maternal MI supplementation (addition of MI in drinking water during pregnancy) (Schneider 2015).

SMIT1 activity is inhibited by lithium, valproate and carbamazepine albeit it does not represent the main mechanism of action of these anti-convulsive agents. Lithium also inhibits the MI-monophosphatase and thus obstructs the enzymatic degradation of inositol triphosphate (IP3) to inositol in the phosphate-phosphoinositide (PIP) cycle. This inhibition may result in reduced availability of the second messengers IP3 and DAG that are derivatives of the PIP cycle, and this action is currently a leading hypothesis regarding lithium's therapeutic and prophylactic effect in affective disorders. Overall mechanisms support the hypothesis that MI depletion is the cause of the way lithium and other mood stabilisers work in treatment of bipolar disorder (Einat et al. 1998).

SMIT2: Expression and Activities

A second Na^+-MI transporter, SMIT2, (also known as SGLT6), has been identified as a Na-coupled *MI* transporter in 2002 by Coady et al. in Xenopus oocytes (Coady et al. 2002).

Analogously to SMIT1, SMIT2 is a member of the SGLT family (table 1) and the *SLC5A* gene family that, in humans, comprises 12 members involved in Na-coupled transport of sugars, iodide, monocarboxylates, and vitamins. These cotransporters seem to operate according to the alternate access mechanism by presenting their binding sites to each side of the membrane and by maintaining a strict stoichiometric ratio between the transported solutes (Wright and Turk 2004). Regarding the stoichiometry for SMIT2, it has been established a 2:1 Na^+: MI ratio (Bourgeois, Coady, and Lapointe 2005).

SMIT2 was shown to be highly expressed in the intestinal epithelium and in proximal tubules, where it mediates the transport of MI. When heterologously expressed in the MDCK renal cell line, SMIT2 is clearly targeted to the apical domain and it mediates the MI uptake in apical membrane of rat small intestine (Bissonnette, Coady, and Lapointe 2004, Aouameur et al. 2007). SMIT2 can be found also in kidney, heart, skeletal muscle, liver and placenta with weak expression in the brain. It transports DCI equally well as MI but does not transport l-fucose.

Based on measurements in oocytes expressing this 66-kDa protein, it has been shown that SMIT2 transports MI with an affinity constant (*K*m) of 120 μM as well as DCI (K_m = 130μM). Indeed, DCI has been used in competitor experiment as a specific inhibitor to distinguish between SMIT1 and SMIT2. Considering that DCI is poorly represented within the plasma (about 0.5 μmol/l), MI is supposed to be the physiological substrate of SMIT2. The affinity for glucose is rather low (K_m ~ 30μM) (Schneider 2015).

Lin et al., by overexpressing SMIT2 cDNA, demonstrated that SMIT2 transports DCI and MI with similar affinity in L6 myoblasts whereas it does not appear to be involved to glucose transport (Lin et al. 2009). Furthermore, DCI transport in L6 myoblasts appeared to be upregulated by insulin probably through an effect on the SMIT2 (Lin et al. 2009). Interestingly, Coady et al. reported that on Xenopus oocytes SMIT2 has a greater affinity for D-glucose than does SMIT1: 50 mM D-glucose produces a current through SMIT2 that is almost half size than the current seen with the same amount of MI less than 25% of the MI current is seen when 50 mM D-glucose is applied to SMIT1 (Coady et al. 2002).

Table 1. The seven SGLT isoforms

Protein name	Human gene name	Predominant substrate	Tissue distribution and cellular expression	Activities
SGLT1	*SLC5A1*	Glucose and galactose	Brush border membranes of enterocytes and in proximal tubules of the kidneys; plasma membranes	Active glucose absorption in intestine and kidneys
SGLT2	*SLC5A2*	Glucose	Kidneys cortex	Glucose reabsorption in tubules
SGLT3	*SLC5A4*	Na^+ (H^+)	Small intestine, skeletal muscle, kidney, uterus and testis; plasma membrane	It is more a glucose "sensor" with an affinity for glucose rather low (Km around 20nM)
SGLT4	*SLC5A8*	Mannose	Small intestine, kidney, liver, lung and brain	
SGLT5	*SLC5A9*	Glucose and galactose	Kidneys	Glucose and galactose reabsorption in tubules
SMIT1	*SLC5A3*	MI	Brain, heart, kidney and lung; plasma membrane	Active co-transport of MI with sodium
SGLT6 (or SMIT2)	*SLC5A10*	MI and DCI	Small intestine and kidney (apical membrane), brain, liver, heart, and lung	Active co-transport with sodium. Rather low affinity for glucose.

HMIT: Expression and Activities

The third MI transporter, HMIT, is H^+-dependent and is predominantly expressed in the brain but very weakly elsewhere (Lahjouji et al. 2007). It is also known as GLUT13 and it was identified in humans and rats in 2001 and it is encoded by the gene SLC2A13 which expression is induced in the brain under hypertonic conditions (Uldry et al. 2001). As the other SLC family member proteins, HMIT is characterized by twelve transmembrane domains, an enlarged loop between the sixth and seventh transmembrane domain and N- and C-terminus located within the cytoplasm.

Rat HMIT was analysed in Xenopus oocytes and shown to be a H^+/MI symporter with a Km of 100 μM. Competitor experiments demonstrated that other inositol isomers such as scyllo-, D-chiro- and muco-inositol are transported by HMIT, while monosaccharides such as glucose or fructose are not.

So far, HMIT localisation is discussed controversially. Uldry et al. showed that HMIT is present in intracellular vesicles but can appear on the cell surface in a P12 cell culture triggered by cell plasma membrane depolarisation, protein kinase C activation or increased intracellular Ca^{2+} concentrations (Uldry et al. 2004). In contrast to this, different experiments observed HMIT localisation only at the Golgi apparatus (Di Daniel et al. 2009). Furthermore, experiments performed by Fu et al. in isolated astrocytes demonstrated that MI uptake is mediated by HMIT under physiologically relevant MI concentrations which points to at least a partial localisation of HMIT within the plasma membrane (Fu et al. 2012).

Independent of its subcellular localization, it is interesting to note that HMIT may play a role in Parkinson disease considering that some studies revealed that SLC2A13 seems to be a Parkinson related gene (Schneider 2015). Furthermore, HMIT can transport IP3, indicating a possible function of this transporter in the intracellular regulation of inositol and phospoinositides by sequestering IP3 into vesicles and thus possibly affecting calcium signaling. This finding may correlate HMIT activity with mood control (Di Daniel et al. 2009).

INOSITOL ORAL INTAKE

Inositol, and in particular MI, is considered an essential dietary factor and its deficiency has been linked to several syndromes.

MI is biosynthesized at tissue levels but an exogenous supplementation by food or dietary supplement may be required to reach higher plasma and tissue concentrations. It is widely used in clinical practice due to its role in different cellular processes including cell proliferation, fertilization and neural activity. Indeed, several clinical trials have already shown that MI plays a crucial role in treating PCOS symptoms such as hyperandrogenism, hyperinsulinaemia and oligo-anovulation. Furthermore, a crucial role of MI in preventing the ovary hyperstimulation syndrome, during assisted reproductive technology protocol, has also been proposed. A number of clinical trials also have suggested that MI administration provides effective results in the treatment of psychiatric disorders such as panic, depression and premenstrual dysphoric disorder (Carlomagno and Unfer 2011).

After oral intake, MI is absorbed in the intestinal tract and then reabsorbed in the renal tubule. Indeed, both the uptake of MI by intestinal fragments and brush border membrane vesicles from rabbit kidney, fish and rats intestine have been studied to some extent. SMIT 2 mediates all the MI uptake at intestine level. As described above, the same transporter is also involved in the intestinal absorption of DCI (Aouameur et al. 2007).

Based on this evidence, it may be speculated that the intake of high doses of DCI may result in an impaired MI absorption.

Pharmacokinetic studies conducted in healthy subjects demonstrated that the supplementation of 2 g MI in powder form allowed to reach a Cmax of about 36.3 μmol/l and a Tmax of about 180 minutes. A double dosage (i.e., the oral supplementation of 4 g of MI) showed a Cmax of about 45 μmol/l and a Tmax of about 122 minutes. Interestingly, the area under the curve (AUC) after administration of 2 g and 4 g of myo-ins in powder seemed to be remarkably similar (Carlomagno et al. 2012).

Recently, Orrù et al. published results from the analysis of MI plasma concentration of 23 healthy volunteers after MI dosing of 2 g (twice a day) or 4 g (once a day) in powder. Data showed that Cmax was dose-dependent (about 35 μmol/l versus 45 μmol/l after the supplementation of 2 g and 4 g of MI respectively) but following 8 hours from MI administration, both dosages reached the baseline plasma concentration. So, the difference between the two PK profiles was only linked to the Cmax but not to the time variable.

The second administration of 2 g MI after 12 hours allowed to obtain another peak, comparable to the first one, guarantying a longer coverage in terms of high MI plasma concentration: this data allows the author to speculate that dividing the daily intake of MI in two doses represents the preferable posology and the best therapeutic approach (Orru et al. 2017).

Interactions between Dietary Intake of Myo-Inositol with Other Substances

Drug-drug interactions (DDIs) are one of the commonest causes of medication error, with a prevalence of 20-40%. In particular, poly-therapy increases the complexity of therapeutic management and thereby the risk of clinically important DDIs, which can induce the development of adverse reactions or reduce the clinical drug efficacy.

DDIs can be classify into two main groups: pharmacokinetic and pharmacodynamic. The first one involves absorption, distribution, metabolism and excretion, whereas the second one may be due to a direct effect at receptorial level, interference with a biological or physiological control process, and an additive/opposed pharmacological effect (Palleria et al. 2013).

In general terms, the pharmacological interactions between molecules (i.e., drugs, dietary supplements, food) have gained wide importance in the clinical practice. These interactions may cause an improved therapeutic effect, or they may increase the risk of side effects, overdoses and reduced efficacy.

With particular reference to Ins, it is necessary to bear in mind that in the market are available many food supplements containing different concentrations of MI, often combined with other molecules such as folic acid, melatonin, glucomannan, sorbitol, sucrose, maltodextrin, vitamin D, cinnamon, alpha lipoic acid, alpha-lactalbumin etc.

For many of these compounds, PK studies and/or data on the possible interactions on MI intestinal absorption are not available.

Specific attention should be paid when MI is administered in combination with other sugary substances or excipients (mono-, di- or poly-saccarides).

Among these, glucomannan is a polysaccharide chain of beta-D-glucose and beta-D-mannose with attached acetyl groups with beta-1,4 linkages. It is a well-known water-soluble fiber that impairs nutrients absorption: due to the lack of beta-1,4-amilase at salivary and pancreatic level, glucomannan passes relatively unchanged into the colon where it is highly fermented by microbiota.

Glucomannan can absorb up to 50 times its weight in water, making it one of the most viscous dietary fibers known and exerting its beneficial effects by promoting satiety and fecal energy loss (Keithley and Swanson 2005).

Considering its mechanism of action, even though glucomannan is generally well tolerated and has a favorable safety profile, additional studies on interference with other molecules, and in particular with Ins, are required.

Maltodextrins are low-sweet saccharide polymers consisting of D-glucose units linked primarily linearly with alpha-1,4 bonds, and more rarely alpha-1,6 bonds and derived by hydrolysis from crops naturally rich in starch.

In drugs or food supplements maltodextrins are used as diluent, as a co-processing excipient and as a coating material to encapsulate nutraceutics such as vitamins.

Digestion of maltodextrins occurs by a pancreatic amylase which is secreted in the small intestine and plays a role in hydrolyzing the α, 1–4 linkages thus forming maltose units. Maltose is either taken up by the gut epithelium directly or further broken down by brush border maltase, resulting in free glucose which is absorbed by active transport (mainly

SGLT1) across the apical membrane of the enterocytes and then across the basal membrane into blood.

Since glucose from digested maltodextrins is rapidly absorbed in the small intestine and subsequently used in metabolism, the increased intake of these substances has raised questions about potential effects on health and possible interactions with the absorption of other nutrients. Indeed, the regular intake of food, drinks or dietary supplements with high levels of refined added CHOs (for instance, maltodextrins) may easily induce a persistent positive energy balance resulting in weight gain, impaired insulin sensitivity, increased blood cholesterol and blood lipids (Hofman, van Buul, and Brouns 2016).

Considering that Ins supplementation is often recommended to treat conditions of insulin resistance or impaired insulin sensitivity, the combined administration with maltodextrins is not clinically supported, rather indeed should be avoided.

Glucose as itself or as the result of digestive process of dietary polysaccharides, is absorbed by enterocytes lining the microvilli of the small intestine (duodenum, jejunum, and ileum). SGLT protein family mediates the uptake of glucose: namely SGLT1 is considered the main transport system across the apical membrane of the enterocytes. On the other side, GLUT2 on the basolateral surface, facilitates the release into the blood stream and, when glucose levels are particularly high, it may facilitate the uptake from the gut lumen (Byers, Howard, and Wang 2017).

Considering that the protein involved in Ins intestinal absorption (SMIT2) shows a low affinity for glucose, some studies investigated the possible interactions between these molecules (Caspary and Crane 1970, Scalera, Natuzzi, and Prezioso 1991). The ability of glucose and MI to inhibit each other uptake has been tested: while 10 mM D-glucose gives a 60% inhibition on the transport of 0.1 mM MI, 10 mM MI has no effect on 0.1 mM D-glucose. This finding leads to the conclusion that MI is not transported by the glucose carrier however a non-competitive mechanism of inhibition can be claimed: it seems that D-glucose binding to the carrier molecule makes the binding of MI more difficult (Scalera, Natuzzi, and Prezioso 1991). Chukwuma et al. demonstrated that oral MI inhibits jejunal glucose absorption and reduces blood glucose increase both in normal and diabetic rat models. According to what the authors observed, these effects may be partly due to delayed gastric emptying and accelerated digesta transit (Chukwuma, Ibrahim, and Islam 2016).

Inositol and Caffeine

Caffeine is involved in MI signalling inhibiting IP3-related calcium channels in neural tissue (Bezprozvanny, Bezprozvannaya, and Ehrlich 1994), thus suggesting the hypothesis of caffeine affecting a biological pathway involved in calcium regulation (Cavalli et al. 2011).

The ryanodine receptors and the IP3 receptors represent the two classes of intracellular Ca^{2+}-release channels: caffeine activates the ryanodine receptor whilst inhibiting the IP3 receptors.

Bezprozvanny et al. showed that the concentration of caffeine typically used to activate ryanodine receptors also decrease the activity of IP3 channels more than 10-fold, definitely resulting in the selective effect of caffeine in inhibition of IP3 generated Ca^{2+} signals in mammalian cells (Bezprozvanny, Bezprozvannaya, and Ehrlich 1994, Hume, McAllister, and Wilson 2009).

It is well known that caffeine interferes with the bioavailability of several drugs (Benvenga et al. 2008) and substances, included inositol.

De Grazia et al. reported that the pharmacokinetic profile of MI, administered in powder form, is negatively affected by the concomitant consumption of one "espresso" coffee. The same study provided evidence that the administration of MI in soft gel form impairs the negative interference of caffeine intake on MI bioavailability (De Grazia et al. 2012).

As both caffeine intake and MI deficiency might increase the risk of occurrence and recurrence for NTDs in experimental models and in humans, the negative correlation between caffeine intake and the bioavailability of MI, further strengthens the hypothesis that its deficiency is a risk factor for NTDs in humans.

Furthermore, MI serum deficiency has been correlated with dysmorphogenesis in cultured rodent embryos and the observation of the prevention of glucose-induced dysmorphogenesis by supplementing MI points to a beneficial effect of MI in embryogenesis. Furthermore, the level of MI in human serum was found critical for embryotrophic activity suggesting that a proper supplementation is imperative in improving of the overall efficiency of clinical in vitro fertilization (Chiu et al. 2002, Chiu and Tam 1992).

Therefore, on the basis of the above reported findings, caffeine consumption during pregnancy should be reduced and, in accordance with the evidence that caffeine interferes with the absorption of MI, the concomitant intake of caffeine and MI should be avoided.

On the other hand, based on what is known, during the periconceptional period a combined supplementation of MI with folic acid should be recommended to prevent the risk of NTDs (Carlomagno et al. 2015, Greene, Leung, and Copp 2017, Cavalli and Copp 2002).

Inositol and α-Lactalbumin

α-Lactalbumin is a molecule belonging to the broader class of milk proteins and it is the second most important protein in whey. It is a small, globular protein composed of 123 amino acid residues with MW of 14.07 kDa in human milk and 14.18 kDa in bovine milk.

α-Lactalbumin is characterized by a wide range of biological activities including enzyme activities, enhancement of nutrient absorption, growth stimulation, anti-inflammatory effects, modulation of the immune system and defence against pathogens.

Monastra et al. recently reported both *in vitro* and *in vivo* data supporting the evidence that the combined administration of α-lactalbumin and MI results in an enhanced MI bioavailability (i.e., intestinal absorption). Indeed, both experiments with human intestinal Caco-2 cells and pharmacokinetic data on healthy subjects were reported.

In vitro, MI absorption in Caco-2 cells was improved in the presence of digested α-lactalbumin being this data associated with an increase in tight junction permeability. Clinically, although peak concentration of plasma MI was similar when MI was administered alone or in combination with lactalbumin (T_{max} ~180 minutes), both the C_{max} and the area under the curve were significantly increased when MI was orally administered in combination with α-lactalbumin (Monastra et al. 2018).

Very interestingly, the combination of MI with α-lactalbumin allowed a significant improvement in the treatment of PCOS women who did not respond to the treatment of MI alone. Three months supplementation of MI plus α-lactalbumin, at the daily dosage of 4000 mg and 100 mg respectively, was correlated with an increase of MI plasma levels and a restoration of ovulation, together with a consistent variation in metabolic and hormone parameters (Montanino Oliva et al. 2018).

CONCLUSION

Independently from the dietary source, Ins absorption takes place at intestinal level and carrier proteins are involved in its uptake. Notably, Ins transport occurs through the apical membranes of intestinal epithelia and renal proxila tube since it is both absorbed from food or dietary supplements and reabsorbed from the renal tubule lumen.

Cosomministration of Ins with other nutrients, excipients and pharmacological active substances may result in both pharmacokinetic and pharmacodynamic interactions giving rise to impaired Ins intestinal absorption, reduced therapeutic effects or, on the contrary, improved bioavailability. At this regard, it is well-known that caffeine interferes with the bioavailability of several drug and substances, included MI.

Indeed, many food supplements containing different concentrations of MI, often combined with other molecules and for many of these formulations, PK studies and/or data on the possible interactions on MI intestinal absorption are not available.

Specific attention should be paid when MI is administered in combination with DCI, considering that the protein transport SMIT2 shows high affinity for both molecules. Furthermore, the co-administration of Ins with other sugary substances or excipients (mono-, di- or poly-saccarides) may results in an impaired absorption due to a non-competitive mechanism of transport inhibition.

On the contrary, recent evidences showed that the combined administration of α-lactalbumin and MI results in an enhanced MI bioavailability and "therapeutic" effect proven on PCOS women classified as resistant to the treatment with MI alone.

On the base of these findings and evidences, it is clear that both PK and PD studies are essential to prove the effectiveness of Ins-based products considering the opportunity or the risk that possible interactions may cause.

References

Aouameur, R., S. Da Cal, P. Bissonnette, M. J. Coady, and J. Y. Lapointe. 2007. "SMIT2 mediates all myo-inositol uptake in apical membranes of rat small intestine." *Am J Physiol Gastrointest Liver Physiol* 293 (6):G1300-7. doi: 10.1152/ajpgi.00422.2007.

Baillargeon, J. P., J. E. Nestler, R. E. Ostlund, T. Apridonidze, and E. Diamanti-Kandarakis. 2008. "Greek hyperinsulinemic women, with or without polycystic ovary syndrome, display altered inositols metabolism." *Hum Reprod* 23 (6):1439-46. doi: 10.1093/humrep/den097.

Benvenga, S., L. Bartolone, M. A. Pappalardo, A. Russo, D. Lapa, G. Giorgianni, G. Saraceno, and F. Trimarchi. 2008. "Altered intestinal absorption of L-thyroxine caused by coffee." *Thyroid* 18 (3):293-301. doi: 10.1089/thy.2007.0222.

Bezprozvanny, I., S. Bezprozvannaya, and B. E. Ehrlich. 1994. "Caffeine-induced inhibition of inositol(1,4,5)-trisphosphate-gated calcium channels from cerebellum." *Mol Biol Cell* 5 (1):97-103.

Bissonnette, P., M. J. Coady, and J. Y. Lapointe. 2004. "Expression of the sodium-myo-inositol cotransporter SMIT2 at the apical membrane of Madin-Darby canine kidney cells." *J Physiol* 558 (Pt 3):759-68. doi: 10.1113/jphysiol.2004.064311.

Bizzarri, M., A. Fuso, S. Dinicola, A. Cucina, and A. Bevilacqua. 2016. "Pharmacodynamics and pharmacokinetics of inositol(s) in health and disease." *Expert Opin Drug Metab Toxicol* 12 (10):1181-96. doi: 10.1080/17425255.2016.1206887.

Bourgeois, F., M. J. Coady, and J. Y. Lapointe. 2005. "Determination of transport stoichiometry for two cation-coupled myo-inositol cotransporters: SMIT2 and HMIT." *J Physiol* 563 (Pt 2):333-43. doi: 10.1113/jphysiol.2004.076679.

Byers, M. S., C. Howard, and X. Wang. 2017. "Avian and Mammalian Facilitative Glucose Transporters." *Microarrays (Basel)* 6 (2). doi: 10.3390/microarrays6020007.

Carlomagno, G., S. De Grazia, V. Unfer, and F. Manna. 2012. "Myo-inositol in a new pharmaceutical form: a step forward to a broader clinical use." *Expert Opin Drug Deliv* 9 (3):267-71. doi: 10.1517/17425247.2012.662953.

Carlomagno, G., S. De Grazia, A. Vaiarelli, and V. Unfer. 2015. *Coffee in health and disease prevention*. Edited by Victor R Preedy: Elsevier.

Carlomagno, G., and V. Unfer. 2011. "Inositol safety: clinical evidences." *Eur Rev Med Pharmacol Sci* 15 (8):931-6.

Caspary, W. F., and R. K. Crane. 1970. "Active transport of myo-inositol and its relation to the sugar transport system in hamster small intestine." *Biochim Biophys Acta* 203 (2):308-16.

Cavalli, P., U. Cavallari, V. Unfer, and G. Tonni. 2011. "Caffeine intake and risk of neural tube defects." *Birth Defects Res A Clin Mol Teratol*. doi: 10.1002/bdra.20739.

Cavalli, P., and A. J. Copp. 2002. "Inositol and folate resistant neural tube defects." *J Med Genet* 39 (2):E5.

Chiu, T. T., M. S. Rogers, E. L. Law, C. M. Briton-Jones, L. P. Cheung, and C. J. Haines. 2002. "Follicular fluid and serum concentrations of myo-inositol in patients undergoing IVF: relationship with oocyte quality." *Hum Reprod* 17 (6):1591-6.

Chiu, T. T., and P. P. Tam. 1992. "A correlation of the outcome of clinical in vitro fertilization with the inositol content and embryotrophic properties of human serum." *J Assist Reprod Genet* 9 (6):524-30.

Chukwuma, C. I., M. A. Ibrahim, and M. S. Islam. 2016. "Myo-inositol inhibits intestinal glucose absorption and promotes muscle glucose uptake: a dual approach study." *J Physiol Biochem* 72 (4):791-801. doi: 10.1007/s13105-016-0517-1.

Coady, M. J., B. Wallendorff, D. G. Gagnon, and J. Y. Lapointe. 2002. "Identification of a novel Na+/myo-inositol cotransporter." *J Biol Chem* 277 (38):35219-24. doi: 10.1074/jbc.M204321200.

De Grazia, S., G. Carlomagno, V. Unfer, and P. Cavalli. 2012. "Myo-inositol soft gel capsules may prevent the risk of coffee-induced neural tube defects." *Expert Opin Drug Deliv* 9 (9):1033-9. doi: 10.1517/17425247.2012.701616.

Di Daniel, E., M. H. Mok, E. Mead, C. Mutinelli, E. Zambello, L. L. Caberlotto, T. J. Pell, C. J. Langmead, A. J. Shah, G. Duddy, J. N. Kew, and P. R. Maycox. 2009. "Evaluation of expression and function of the H+/myo-inositol transporter HMIT." *BMC Cell Biol* 10:54. doi: 10.1186/1471-2121-10-54.

Einat, H., O. Kofman, O. Itkin, R. J. Lewitan, and R. H. Belmaker. 1998. "Augmentation of lithium's behavioral effect by inositol uptake inhibitors." *J Neural Transm (Vienna)* 105 (1):31-8. doi: 10.1007/s007020050035.

Fu, H., B. Li, L. Hertz, and L. Peng. 2012. "Contributions in astrocytes of SMIT1/2 and HMIT to myo-inositol uptake at different concentrations and pH." *Neurochem Int* 61 (2):187-94. doi: 10.1016/j.neuint. 2012.04.010.

Greene, N. D., K. Y. Leung, and A. J. Copp. 2017. "Inositol, neural tube closure and the prevention of neural tube defects." *Birth Defects Res* 109 (2):68-80. doi: 10.1002/bdra.23533.

Hofman, D. L., V. J. van Buul, and F. J. Brouns. 2016. "Nutrition, Health, and Regulatory Aspects of Digestible Maltodextrins." *Crit Rev Food Sci Nutr* 56 (12):2091-100. doi: 10.1080/10408398.2014.940415.

Hume, J. R., C. E. McAllister, and S. M. Wilson. 2009. "Caffeine inhibits InsP3 responses and capacitative calcium entry in canine pulmonary arterial smooth muscle cells." *Vascul Pharmacol* 50 (3-4):89-97. doi: S1537-1891(08)00139-0 [pii] 10.1016/j.vph.2008.11.001.

Keithley, J., and B. Swanson. 2005. "Glucomannan and obesity: a critical review." *Altern Ther Health Med* 11 (6):30-4.

Kwon, H. M., A. Yamauchi, S. Uchida, A. S. Preston, A. Garcia-Perez, M. B. Burg, and J. S. Handler. 1992. "Cloning of the cDNa for a Na+/myo-inositol cotransporter, a hypertonicity stress protein." *J Biol Chem* 267 (9):6297-301.

Lahjouji, K., R. Aouameur, P. Bissonnette, M. J. Coady, D. G. Bichet, and J. Y. Lapointe. 2007. "Expression and functionality of the Na+/myo-inositol cotransporter SMIT2 in rabbit kidney." *Biochim Biophys Acta* 1768 (5):1154-9. doi: 10.1016/j.bbamem.2007.01.007.

Lin, X., L. Ma, R. L. Fitzgerald, and R. E. Ostlund, Jr. 2009. "Human sodium/inositol cotransporter 2 (SMIT2) transports inositols but not glucose in L6 cells." *Arch Biochem Biophys* 481 (2):197-201. doi: 10.1016/j.abb.2008.11.008.

Monastra, G., S. Ferruzza, Y. Sambuy, G. Ranaldi, and D. Ferrari. 2018. "Alpha-lactalbumin effect on myo-inositol intestinal absorption: in vivo and in vitro." *Curr Drug Deliv*. doi: 10.2174/1567201815666180509102641.

Montanino Oliva, M., G. Buonomo, M. Calcagno, and V. Unfer. 2018. "Effects of myo-inositol plus alpha-lactalbumin in myo-inositol-resistant PCOS women." *J Ovarian Res* 11 (1):38. doi: 10.1186/s13048-018-0411-2.

Orru, B., R. Circo, P. Logoteta, S. Petousis, and G. Carlomagno. 2017. "Finding the best therapeutic approach for PCOS: the importance of inositol(s) bioavailability." *Eur Rev Med Pharmacol Sci* 21 (2 Suppl):83-88.

Palleria, C., A. Di Paolo, C. Giofre, C. Caglioti, G. Leuzzi, A. Siniscalchi, G. De Sarro, and L. Gallelli. 2013. "Pharmacokinetic drug-drug interaction and their implication in clinical management." *J Res Med Sci* 18 (7):601-10.

Scalera, V., D. Natuzzi, and G. Prezioso. 1991. "myo-inositol transport in rat intestinal brush border membrane vesicles, and its inhibition by D-glucose." *Biochim Biophys Acta* 1062 (2):187-92.

Schneider, S. 2015. "Inositol transport proteins." *FEBS Lett* 589 (10):1049-58. doi: 10.1016/j.febslet.2015.03.012.

Uldry, M., M. Ibberson, J. D. Horisberger, J. Y. Chatton, B. M. Riederer, and B. Thorens. 2001. "Identification of a mammalian H(+)-myo-inositol symporter expressed predominantly in the brain." *EMBO J* 20 (16):4467-77. doi: 10.1093/emboj/20.16.4467.

Uldry, M., P. Steiner, M. G. Zurich, P. Beguin, H. Hirling, W. Dolci, and B. Thorens. 2004. "Regulated exocytosis of an H+/myo-inositol symporter at synapses and growth cones." *EMBO J* 23 (3):531-40. doi: 10.1038/sj.emboj.7600072.

Unfer, V. 2018. "Use of alpha-lactalbumin for the management of PCOS in inositols resistant women." *Eur Rev Med Pharmacol Sci* 22 (7):1873-1874. doi: 10.26355/eurrev_201804_14705.

Van Steenbergen, A., M. Balteau, A. Ginion, L. Ferte, S. Battault, C. M. Ravenstein, J. L. Balligand, E. P. Daskalopoulos, P. Gilon, F. Despa, S. Despa, J. L. Vanoverschelde, S. Horman, H. Koepsell, G. Berry, L. Hue, L. Bertrand, and C. Beauloye. 2017. "Sodium-myoinositol cotransporter-1, SMIT1, mediates the production of reactive oxygen species induced by hyperglycemia in the heart." *Sci Rep* 7:41166. doi: 10.1038/srep41166.

Wright, E. M., and E. Turk. 2004. "The sodium/glucose cotransport family SLC5." *Pflugers Arch* 447 (5):510-8. doi: 10.1007/s00424-003-1063-6.

ABOUT THE EDITOR

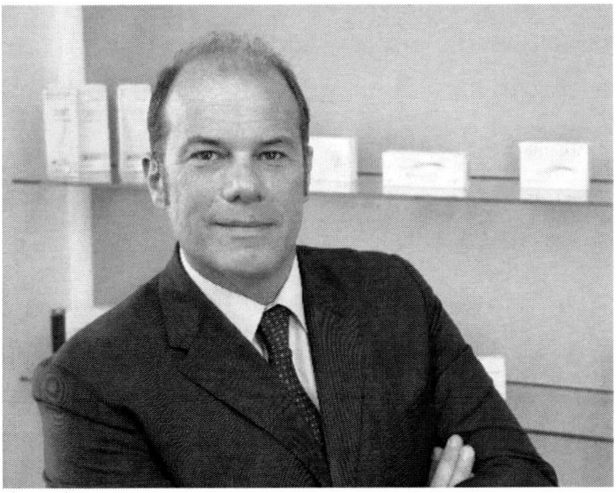

Vittorio Unfer, MD, was born in Rome on October 12, 1963 where he currently lives and works as an Obstetrics and Gynaecology Specialist, researcher and university lecturer.

He graduated with honors in 1991 in Medicine and Surgery at the Faculty of Medicine of Sapienza University of Rome, successively he decided to enroll to the specialization in obstetrics and gynecology at the II Clinical Institute of Obstetrics and Gynaecology of Policlinico Umberto I in Rome, obtaining a score of 70 out of 70 with honors in 1995.

Academic Activities

Currently, Vittorio Unfer is Lecturer at the Department of Experimental Medicine, Sapienza University (Rome, Italy).

He was Master Professor in "Unconventional Medicine in assisting Obstetrics and Nursing Autonomy and midwife in the management of pregnancy, childbirth and postpartum low risk" at the Faculty of Medicine, University of Modena and Reggio Emilia.

He is also Full Professor at the University IPUS (Advanced Training Institute) of Chiasso, Switzerland.

In 2010 he was appointed as a lecturer in Endocrinology childhood, adolescence and women at the University Master's Degree, School of Specialization in Endocrinology, Degree Course in Medicine and Surgery of University of Messina.

From 2008 to 2011 he teaches nutrition and food disease in pregnancy at the School of Specialization in Gynaecology and Obstetrics, Degree Course in Obstetrics, University of Perugia.

In the Academic Year 2001-2002 is a Professor of Health Statistics at the Department of Gynaecological Sciences, Perinatal and Child-care , Degree Course in Obstetrics, Sapienza University of Rome.

From 1999 to 2000 he works as a Professor of Forensic Medicine at the Department of Gynaecological Sciences, Perinatal and Child-care, Degree Course in Obstetrics, Sapienza University of Rome.

Research Activities

He is also the author of numerous publications: over 50 international journals, more than 90 publications in national magazines, over 10 monographs and edited works, more than 100 abstracts in national and international periodicals, among the most important and recent is relevant to mention:

1. Unfer V, Facchinetti F, Orrù B, Giordani B, Nestler J. Myo-inositol effects in women with PCOS: a meta-analysis of randomized controlled trials. *Endocr Connect.* 2017 Nov;6(8):647-658.

2. Unfer V, Nestler JE, Kamenov ZA, Prapas N, Facchinetti F. Effects of Inositol(s) in Women with PCOS: A Systematic Review of Randomized Controlled Trials. *International Journal of Endocrinology.* Volume 2016, Article ID 1849162.
3. Gullo G, Carlomagno G, Unfer V, D'Anna R. "Myo-inositol: from induction of ovulation to menopausal disorder management". *Minerva Ginecol*. 2015 Oct.
4. Santamaria A, Corrado F, Baviera G, Carlomagno G, Unfer V, D'anna R. "Second trimester amniotic fluid myo-inositol concentrations in women later developing gestational diabetes mellitus or pregnancy-induced hypertension". *J Matern Fetal Neonatal Med.* Epub 2015 Sep 12.
5. Nestler JE, Unfer V., "Reflections on inositol(s) for PCOS therapy: steps toward success". *Gynecol Endocrinol.* 2015 Jul.
6. Carlomagno G, Unfer V, Benvenga S, Nestler JE. "Myo-inositol: with or without". *Endocr J.* 2015;62(3):297-8. doi: 10.1507/endocrj.EJ14-0566. Epub 2015 Jan 31.
7. Costantino M, Guaraldi C, Costantino D, De Grazia S, Unfer V. "Peripheral neuropathy in obstetrics: efficacy and safety of α-lipoic acid supplementation" *Eur Rev Med Pharmacol Sci.* 2014;18(18):2766-71. Review.
8. Dinicola S, Chiu TT, Unfer V, Carlomagno G, Bizzarri M. "The rationale of the myo-inositol and D-chiro-inositol combined treatment for polycystic ovary syndrome". *J Clin Pharmacol.* 2014 Oct;54(10):1079-92. doi: 10.1002/jcph.362. Epub 2014 Jul 18. Review.
9. Santamaria A, Corrado F, Interdonato ML, Baviera G, Carlomagno G, Cavalli P, Unfer V, D'Anna R. "Myo-inositol in Down syndrome amniotic fluid. A case-control study". *Prenat Diagn.* 2014 Sep;34(9):917-8. doi: 10.1002/pd.4398. Epub 2014 Jul 5.
10. Unfer V, Porcaro G. "Updates on the myo-inositol plus D-chiro-inositol combined therapy in polycystic ovary syndrome". *Expert Rev Clin Pharmacol.* 2014 Sep;7(5):623-31. doi: 10.1586/17512433.2014.925795. Epub 2014 Jun 5. Review.

11. Unfer V, Carlomagno G, Papaleo E, Vailati S, Candiani M, Baillargeon JP. "Hyperinsulinemia Alters Myo-inositol to d-chiroinositol Ratio in the Follicular Fluid of Patients with PCOS". *Reprod Sci.* 2014 Feb 4;21(7):854-858. [Epub ahead of print].
12. Della Vella B, Unfer V, Nania C, Borgia ML, Saraceno A, Minozzi M. "Hereditary hemorrhagic telangiectasia and pregnancy: case report". *Eur Rev Med Pharmacol Sci.* 2012 Jul;16(7):986-9.

In 2005 he contributed to the drafting of the Treaty of Gynaecology and Obstetrics published by Verduci and currently is still an active member of Verduci ECM Scientific Committee.

The intensive research in recent times of Professor Vittorio Unfer is connected to aspects of nutrition and use of food supplements in obstetrics and gynaecology clinical practice.

In the academic sector, Professor Vittorio Unfer participated in many other important scientific research focused on the morphofunctional study of uterine contractile activity with previous uterine scar, the triggering mechanisms of labor, the treatment of the threatened miscarriage abortion and prevention of preterm labor in high-risk patients, the treatment of hypogonadotropic male hypogonadism with FSH, and several in-depth and comparative experimentations on the fetal maturity.

It is few years that the scientific contribution of Professor Vittorio Unfer is related to the investigations focused on PCOS (polycystic ovary syndrome) and in particular on the role of second messengers in ovarian function.

Professor Vittorio Unfer resulted to be the first promoter of the use of myo-inositol in the treatment for polycystic ovary syndrome; his in-depth research pointed out the beneficial effects of the myo-inositol molecule on ovarian function and metabolic parameters.

These results were highly appreciated by the international community due to the findings of Professor Vittorio Unfer. Today the treatment with myo-inositol for women with PCOS is adopted in more than 36 countries.

Private Activities

Professor Vittorio Unfer currently is the Medical Director and Gynaecologist at “A.G.UN.CO. – Studi Polimedici Specialistici”.

He is in charge as President of the Pharmaceutical Society Lo.Li Pharma Ltd, Chairman of the Board of Lo.Li Pharma International Ltd. As well as Chairman of the Board of Farmares Ltd, research and development company.

Professor Vittorio Unfer, moreover holds the position of Vice President of SIFIPsi (Italian Society of Phytotherapy and supplements in Psychopathology), he is member of the Pharmaceutical Society Bioitalia Ltd, Co- founder of ISCHOM (International Society of Chocolate, Cocoa in Medicine) and is Past-President of SIFIOG, Italian Society of Phytotherapy and supplements in Obstetrics and Gynaecology.

Since 1995 he attended more than 25 training courses to enhance his professional skills.

He participated as a speaker in many national and international conferences in the Endocrinology Gynaecology and Obstetrics fields.

Lately Professor Vittorio Unfer has been guest on various TV shows and radio broadcasting programs as expert on issues related to infertility and PCOS, such as "Sulle Ali della Salute”, " Medicina, Salute e Benessere”, “Mattino Cinque” on Channel 5, Tg Norba 24 and Sky Channel 913.

Contact

Email: vunfer@gmail.com

INDEX

#

α

β

A

B

C

D

E

F

L

M

N

O

P

R

S

T

U